ADVANCE PRAISE

I presented Dr Balesh with The Day of Compassion Award and was amazed when I heard about her rural practice and the difference she was making in thousands of lives.

An eye-opener, this book will educate and amuse you. Honestly written, it is about how a young doctor changed the healthcare scene in a rural population.

Four decades of a rural practice, five generations of patients, watching a third-world country wake up to globalisation, new farmland wealth and the highs and lows of human behaviour, Balesh has seen it all. Masterfully crafted, the book holds you spellbound till the last page leaving you wanting for more.

These stories have never been heard and told with so much candidness. The glimmer of hope in poverty, the poignancy of desperation and acceptance in the face of death, all of this is experienced in this sobering, yet elegant book.

Dr Philip Zimbardo
Professor Emeritus of Psychology, Stanford University

The Reluctant Doctor is an attempt by a doctor, a lady, belonging to a class which has the privilege of options, choices and luxuries to share her personal thoughts and challenges while passing through her professional journey, Dr Balesh has overcome all challenges and done a wonderful job of it. The book is a compelling account, honest and insightful; it chronicles tales of the effects of liberalisation and surplus wealth on an unprepared rural population. These tales span thirty-eight unhurried years as each fascinating story unfolds and transports us to an unfamiliar world. A young doctor was able to change the lives of thousands of patients who streamed into her small clinic, treating not only physical disease but solving psychological, financial, marital and adolescent issues. Extremely enjoyable and readable for both doctors and the common man, who can relate to the situations and environment and pick up leads to apply in their own lives.
A must read for all.

Dr GS Grewal

President, Indian Medical Association, New Delhi

THE RELUCTANT DOCTOR

THE RELUCTANT DOCTOR

STILETTOS TO STETHOSCOPE

TRUE STORIES FROM INSIDE A CLINIC

BALESH JINDAL

Vitasta

Published by
Renu Kaul Verma
Vitasta Publishing Pvt Ltd
4348/4C, Ansari Road, Daryaganj
New Delhi-110 002
info@vitastapublishing.com

ISBN 978-93-90961-74-0

First Edition 2022

MRP ₹ 495

Edited by Veena Batra
Layout and Cover design by Somesh Kumar Mishra
Printed by Thomson Press India Ltd.

CONTENTS

Acknowledgements *ix*

Preface *xi*

Foreword *xiii*

Why are these Stories Important? *xvii*

The Beginning 1

The Uncertain Doctor 27

After the Accident 43

Kalawati Saran Children's Hospital (KWSCH) 1982 48

All about Radiology 60

Learning and Unlearning 1983-2020 67

Quacksalvers and Voodoo 81

Bijwasan 96

My Clinic 109

Was this a Miracle? 125
The Reluctant Gynaecologist 133
All about Bad Milk 146
Histories and Stories 149
The Girl's Period or a Curse 156
Travelling along NH 8 163
Bijwasan and the Harvest Season 176
Mornings at the Railway Track 189
The People of Rajokri 195
Then Came Maggi Noodles and More 212
Early 2000s and Sackfuls of Money 221
Boyfriend Season 237
Boys will be Boys 243
The Second New Bride 248
The Big Fat Indian Family 255

ACKNOWLEDGEMENTS

I HAVE TO thank my father for his vision and for setting me on this truly incredible journey of a lifetime. I thank my mother for her silent support behind the curtains. I learnt my life lessons from her silences.

I am grateful to Rattan, my husband, for always having my back and for his endless guidance as I floundered along learning the finer nuances of being a doctor.

I need to thank Rahul and Mehul for their constant encouragement and their gift of a beautiful writing table where I spent the entire year of the first Covid wave writing and rewriting this book. If it were not for them this book would still be on my bucket list waiting.

I thank all my patients who stepped inside my clinic to enrich me and to let me learn from them. I am grateful to them for being a part of my journey for without them there would have been no journey. I am truly overwhelmed by the trust and the affection that they showered on me. Without the trust of my patients I wouldn't be half the person that I am today. I assure all of them that I have taken utmost care to protect their identity and not a single one of them can be identified.

PREFACE

THE RELUCTANT DOCTOR takes the reader on a forty-year biographical journey that is honest and vulnerable—vulnerable because all emotions have been laid bare with no safety nets. These are stories of hope, desolation, decadence and tragedy. Yet, they inspire because even when there was no hope in sight, I continued trudging along and doing what I thought had to be done. Doing so left me with so many questions that confounded me.

How much compassion is good enough? I used to wonder.

If one's own child has a fever, isn't it best for a doctor to steer clear of her patients and tend to her own child?

Is it right for a doctor to get so involved with her patients that she forgets her child's bad grades, tantrums and school functions?

Is it appropriate for a doctor to feel so empathetic towards her patients that she has no time to empathise with her own family?

What is too little and too much caring?

When does empathy become pathological?

This is the story of a rural medical practice I built from a small guardroom with just a small table and chair. I stare at the pages before me, unable to transfer a single thought as I am faced with a paucity of words that lay unused for four decades, drowned in the mundane. The narration may lack technique but the stories are vivid and real.

The Reluctant Doctor is a memoir, but at the same time it's not just a personal memoir. It's a socioeconomic commentary witnessed by a person who just happened to be there for almost four decades. The book chronicles tales about the way society moved with the advent of new wealth, exposure to modernity, and westernisation of an emerging economy.

Each patient influenced me like no other; I internalised and lived thousands of those lives as my own. I felt their agony as my own and their stories went home with me and kept me awake at night. The boundaries of their lives merged with mine till I was one with them.

From a callow doctor who regretted the day she set foot in Kapashera, I found peace and gratification in the rural medical practice. I like to believe that I left indelible footsteps as I tread on this unglamorous path to leave the world a better place.

Balesh Jindal

FOREWORD

SEVERAL YEARS AGO, much before I got to know Balesh Jindal—doctor, painter and now writer—I lived in Gurgaon for a while, between postings. Virtually every day on my way to and from work, I'd drive past a corner building bang on a busy crossroads, bearing the name 'Dr Jindal's Clinic'. As I waited for the lights to change, I would idly visualise the physician inside as a ponderous, bespectacled gentleman dispensing, with rough kindness, advice, admonishment, prescriptions and strips of specimen medicines amongst hordes of ardent patients.

You can imagine my surprise, hence, when I met Balesh for the first time in her alternative avatar of renowned artist and learnt that *she* was the Dr Jindal presiding over the clinic that had become, for a time, such a quintessential part of my travel landscape! Warmly feminine, elegant, soft-spoken and dreamy-eyed, she couldn't have been more different from the middle-aged doctor with salt-and-pepper hair that I'd conjured in my mind. Or even, to be truthful, from the stern, no-nonsense woman I could sort of see running a clinic in a place like Kapashera—that blade of dense, semi-rural earthiness slashing through the belly of the glamourous, glittery uber-urban sprawl of modern Gurugram. In the days when Balesh decided to set up her clinic in this part of the city, things were even more primitive, as she shares with us in this gritty book that doesn't shy away from the dirt and grime, the tears and the blood she witnessed and experienced. Gurgaon barely qualified as a town then—much farther from Delhi in terms of awareness than it was in kilometres—and nobody had even heard of the dusty little village of Kapashera.

For a gently brought up young woman belonging to a well-heeled family, and a fresh medical graduate at that, it must have been a nightmare of monumental proportions to set up shop in a place like that and deal with a half-hostile, half-indifferent and fully patriarchal society in which women's health was the last priority and a female doctor was a joke. I have no idea what her endlessly indulgent father was thinking when he gently nudged her into that clinic in Kapashera, but boy, did he create a person, a daughter and a doctor he could be proud of!

As you walk with Balesh through the heart-rending cases, the appalling circumstances, the terrible crimes and their monstrous perpetrators, the emotional trauma of the girls and women she treated—and by extension of Balesh herself—you wonder how she survived all that. Your admiration grows as you understand that she didn't merely survive; she persisted and broke through gender-barriers and rural-urban divides, making a place for herself and creating space for her work. She saved the lives and sanity of countless women while herself evolving into a compassionate human being and healer despite the horrors she witnessed and dealt with. Not letting the scars on your psyche mar your behaviour and responses is an achievement in itself, but to actually emerge stronger and brighter from that ordeal, as Balesh did, defines and refines the very metal of your soul.

Balesh's book is a saga of tragedy, courage, grit, determination and rage. May you derive inspiration from it to do what you can to change the world around you in small ways and big. Both are equally important.

Sangeeta Bahadur
High Commissioner of India to the Republic of Malta
Author, *The Kaal Trilogy*

WHY ARE THESE STORIES IMPORTANT?

I SAW THE advent of violence and sex in movies reflected in real life with uncanny accuracy; almost none of it was ever reported. *There are no records of these but someone has to account for them.*

As dating became an option, unwanted pregnancies flooded the clinic in the eighties.

Someone has to hear the tales of woe of these simple village girls who got churned ruthlessly in the modernisation wave.

School boys could be seen injecting drugs in their veins in every back alley.

The lost lives of these little boys have to be acknowledged for they didn't know better.

The redness or blueness on the face, neck and abdomen screamed of physical abuse. None of the women would ever admit they had been beaten. They were silent.

These are stories of silence. When the silence is so deafening, it has to be heard.

I saw the bride that was pushed into the flames after being doused with kerosene brought to my clinic with burns so fresh that I saw her clothes fused with her flesh. *How do I efface those dying eyes? How do I erase the pain that I saw in them?*

The cold-blooded murder of Sikhs in 1984 when the Indian prime minister was assassinated by her guard happened right before me. I heard the mob had tied a whole family to a post and burnt them alive along with women and small children. *The story of this family needs vindication. It has to be read.*

I concede that life has enough drama of its own without us creating anymore, so no dramatic additives were needed for this narrative. I have indulged in the writer's license to change the chronological order. Decades have gotten jumbled up. Families are fitted like jigsaw puzzles to protect the privacy of the individuals. Yet, each incident is like a single piece of the whole puzzle, where each patient is intrinsic to the whole story yet cannot be identified on his own. As you go through this memoir, I ask you not to judge me as a person, dissect my personal life or try to relate any characters to anyone in real life, for that will not be correct. Each incident or person is like a sparrow that has been taken from different summers and different gardens. The completeness lies only in my mind.

CHAPTER ONE

The Beginning

IT ALL STARTED IN 1983. Although I was officially a fully-trained doctor, I had no plans for myself. All my plans hinged on my husband's as he had left for England soon after we were married. Being at a loose end, I twiddled my thumbs and studied for post-graduation with a heedless mind as my dreams were now set in England where I hoped to join my husband. I had decided that I would specialise in Paediatrics. Thoughts of strolling around Trafalgar square, gazing at the enchanting Thames and browsing around Borough Street filled my mind. To me it seemed perfectly okay if I chose to keep myself occupied for the time being, with the leisurely activity of being lonely and idle, even as the literal heavyweights like *Grey's Anatomy* and *Bailey's & Love's Surgery* lay on my table. Seeing the intimidating books, the family presumed that I was preparing for the MD entrance exam but I was busy with my reveries that took me walking on London roads.

The family business was doing well but I was too busy with other avenues of youthful pursuits to notice the ascent of the business. It was the ancillaries of this newly-acquired wealth that were more noticeable to my busy, erudite mind. There were a lot of new clothes, shoes, parties and cars for all of us. My brothers and I started to take this new affluence for granted. I noticed in passing that Mother looked pretty in her beautiful new chiffon sarees with diamonds in her ears. A bright red sedan graced our driveway.

The 8-acre farm that Father had bought and started to develop into a liveable, dreamlike farmhouse was in a rural suburb called Kapashera, an hour's drive from Delhi. In today's day and age, owning a farmhouse is a common thing amongst the wealthy, but in 1982 it was a rarity. I recall our family having endless conversations and debates, with varying degrees of intensity, at most mealtimes, about the beauty of the farm. It became Father's dream project and the unpretentious joy that would radiate from his face as he spoke about it was infectious and drenched everyone in its embrace.

Little did I know then that my fate was inexorably intertwined with that of the farm and that it would be my *karma bhoomi* (place of action) for the entirety of my career. It would be where I would grow and mature as a person and find a calling that was preordained. But that would be running ahead of the story....

However, in the midst of the flurry of buying new cars and expanding the business, Father must have noticed me twiddling my thumbs. One day, quite out of context, at the breakfast table, he looked at me and suggested innocuously, "Why don't you come to the farm with me every morning?"

Then he continued looking at his plate in pretended absorption with his toast.

"Why? What would I do there?" I said in a perfectly calculated disinterested tone, for I recognised a bait when I saw one. I had read enough psychology to know how to disengage and transfer sudden interest away from oneself. I too continued eating my toast. He did not take my pretended disinterest seriously enough. "My farm labourers keep getting sick and miss out on a lot of work. You could treat them for fevers at least," he said without a comment about my obvious disinterest.

"I don't know how to treat fevers," I said warily. I knew how to put my foot down. I raised the intensity of the perfectly bored look and got up to walk away from the breakfast table, leaving my toast unfinished to show my displeasure. I was confident that I could manage Father as I was his 'doted upon' daughter. Wasn't I? I just had to find an opportune moment to make my decision known. I knew from experience that he always came around to whatever I wanted. There was no way that he would want me to practise in Kapashera. He was the one who indulged me with the best clothes, cars and spending money.

He knew I was too good for Kapashera.

"Oh, everyone can treat fevers. Even I can!" he said in a gentle but firm tone that I should have recognised; it meant that a "no" was not an option. I needed to deal with this cautiously.

"You can come and give them just a few tablets for a few days." I could gauge that this was becoming delicate ground and I didn't know how to wriggle out of the situation.

"But I don't know what to give them. We were not taught

how to give tablets," I protested and looked suitably disconcerted and pitiable. Maybe he would take pity on his dear daughter and his heart would melt at my tone and agonised look. He always came around whenever I used that face and tone.

"What did they teach you for six years?" he continued, sounding peeved. This meant that he could see through my dallying. None of my calculated strategies worked that morning and I was surprised at his persistence that day because I had not experienced this attitude before. He always gave in to anything I wished for. He definitely had a game plan there.

Well, tomorrow is another day, I thought. I was optimistic. He may change his mind later, I hoped fervently. The next morning there was no such luck. Sure enough, Father turned up at my place in his car. Without a fuss, I sat in the car and we were soon on our way to this faraway place called Kapashera.

I had used up all the tricks in my ammunition to put him off his plan but he seemed determined. I wasn't one to give up easily and thought that I would give it another try. As the car whirred and zoomed, I said, "I want to go to England, you know that." I spoke in a perfectly low voice laced with emotion and even managed a moist eye. This tone was a sure winner, I knew. There was no response and he looked straight ahead.

I could not fathom what had got into my father as none of my strategies seemed to be working. There seemed to be no deterrent to his resolve. How wrong he was to presume that I would treat his labourers. He would soon realise his folly, I preened. Didn't I always have my way? Surely, this was just a day's indulgence. It would do me no harm to humour him.

"You can leave whenever you want," he said without taking his eyes off the road. Now that was a comforting thought.

Of course I will leave, my mind thought saucily.

The narrow road twisted and turned endlessly and became narrower with each passing metre, which contrasted with the straight roads in the heart of Delhi—roads that I was familiar with. "You will like it, I know," he said looking at the road ahead.

How wrong he was! Like it! Never! Look at the stupid, broken road!

As we crossed the main habitation of Delhi, the wide stretch of the airport road became visible and suddenly the highway became prettier. Mustard fields lay spread on both sides. They were a vision in deep yellow as it was May, the flowering season. I was so enamoured by the sudden appearance of this splash of yellow that I forgot to be grumpy. For a moment it seemed like a dream. Remembering that it was imperative to maintain my unhappy demeanour for Father, lowering my guard even for a moment would be sacrilegious. Grumpiness and displeasure at all times were my strongest armaments. The mustard fields received silent admiration. The ethereal beauty of the fields was the only redeeming factor on that summer's day. The tiny flowers looked like a sea of yellow bobbing heads at a winter carnival. The fields spread out so far that they appeared to be a big yellow sheet nailed to the azure horizon, and they looked an extension of the sky itself. The sunlight drenched the fields generously till they were saturated with a dust of gold. The sight held me spellbound, even as I rued the drive.

The long car ride continued in silence which was largely comfortable as I was busy with the histrionics of my mind, and probably Father too was planning his next move.

There were no highways at that time yet this winding

country road was called NH8 (National Highway 8) for nothing. Probably it was in anticipation of the grand eight-lane expressway that it was destined to become decades later. That day it was just a muddy, village path deviously embedded with crater-like depressions. I sulked and became sulkier by the mile. My convictions became stronger about the foolhardiness of the decision to take me to the farm. I wanted to twiddle my thumbs just a bit longer till my husband returned with his exciting plans. We would fly to London and Kapashera would be left far behind.

After an endless drive, the car stopped in front of a yellow iron gate. I scanned the area squinting my eyes as the overhead sun blazed with a mocking brightness. The scanning of the farm was aptly covert to show my obvious disinterest and to convince Father about my rejection of his idea. I could see a vast stretch of land that lay before me. Eight acres meant that it rolled into the horizon and one could not see where it ended. The smile and pride on my father's face belied any doubts that it was indeed The Farm, where we had finally arrived.

This was the day in May of 1983 that changed my life forever.

I remember being so incredibly distraught at the thought of treating my father's farm labourers, that I missed the beauty of the virgin farm. Later, as I wrote *The Reluctant Doctor*, the first look of the farm surfaced in its freshness and clarity. As I looked beyond the yellow gate, I saw some very tall poplar trees that were years old. They swayed with the summer breeze in rhythm. I hadn't seen this in a long time because rambling along hospital corridors had taken up all of my time for the past seven years. Their coin-like leaves frolicked naughtily against the deep blue sky. Below the rows of tall poplar trees, the thick, tall and long blades of grass rustled in the soft wind. As tall as the whitewashed, five-feet boundary wall they swayed like waves and caressed the white wall seductively. I recognised one of the tall grasses. They were maize plants as baby cobs lay hidden amongst the whorls of spade-like leaves. The rest of the grass was unidentifiable to my untrained eye. Must be a wild variety, I thought.

I shook myself from the reverie. I didn't care what they were; it wouldn't have mattered even if there were apples growing on the grasses, as there were far more pressing problems to burden my mind with. The rows of small saplings of silver oaks along the main path, looking really pretty, caught my eye again. Father must have planted these during his first month at the farm. Those silver oak saplings filled my heart with sadness later over the years. After a decade and the decades that came after, they soared tall and majestic, frolicking in the skies and never failed to remind me of Father.

Even with my grumpy and biased vision, there was no way that I could fail to notice that Father had done extensive landscaping. A pretty hillock rose gently in the distance with verdant grass smiling indolently; a small hibiscus about to flower sat pretty on it. Father had marked out meticulous beds, labelled neatly for roses, gladioli, sunflowers and pretty larkspurs. I could see two large lawns. "These are for parties," he said. I followed him mindlessly around the farm looking and stopping at various places. Tiny tufts of smooth Mexican grass had been planted on these lawns. By monsoon, these would be lush as the soft grass had already started to spread its feet flirtatiously on the sprawling lawns. Following my appreciative gaze at the plants and flower beds, Father explained, "Just behind these gardens will be the house where we will live; it will have a big swimming pool. Come look, I will show you, each bedroom has its own balcony...for morning tea," his voice trailed off as he cast a pensive look towards where the house would be. His look seemed stained with a little sadness. I couldn't help noticing it and a feeling of an unfamiliar sadness overcame me too. Shaking myself out of the sad stupor I kept up the pretense of disinterest for my displeasure had to be known clearly. Faltering in the mission was not the goal.

However, his cheerful voice tinged with hints of wistfulness and sadness still rings clear in my mind as I reminisce about that summer day. I wish I had been more responsive to him and not marred his enthusiasm with my churlish behaviour. There have been many times when his sad look at the farm that day still rankles. Why was he sad that day?

Did that faraway look have a meaning? Could he sense the future?

Did he have a foreboding?

"The vegetable farm will be on this side," he explained with an enthusiastic flick of his right hand.

It was important to look away from him at this point, refusing to let him think that treating his labourers was an option for me. Just one genial expression on my face could turn treacherous and spoil my case. "All this land will be yours," he was saying with a sweep of his hand across the acres of farmland that lay behind the clinic.

I am so much better than this, I kept repeating to myself indignantly. Just the thought of this rural practice made my stomach churn with anxiety. It has to be temporary, I reassured myself. Father can't be serious. After all, he knows that I don't belong here. Just a day or two at the farm ought to settle his enthusiasm, and would do no harm.

Father walked further and called out loudly, "Baburam, Baburam, come here."

A dark, scraggly Baburam came bounding towards us like an excited sheep dog. He would have wagged his tail, had he one. He was clad in a white, grimy loincloth and his ribbed torso was dark and scrawny. It glistened with sweat. His teeth flashed bright in his dark face as he greeted us with a toothy smile. He smiled at me. "Namaste," he said, adding "madam," as an afterthought. I could see he was a bit hesitant to speak with me and rather shy. He smiled and kept that smile plastered the entire time, for lack of any other expression, I assumed.

When one has nothing much to do, one can only smile.

"What is your problem?" Father asked him, exuding more of a swaggering confidence than I felt—a confidence apt for a doctor's father, I mused. "Here is a doctor. You can tell her all your problems." Suddenly both men were looking at me and the searchlight was focused on my face. I shrank further into my frame hoping to become invisible.

I was too new a doctor to consider myself a real one.

The nomenclature of Doctor sounded unfamiliar to my ears, even after completing the mandatory six month rural posting designed to get the feel of the real world and real patients. The place we were posted to was a tiny Government Primary Health Centre in Najafgarh. These centres were the backbone of the free medical care provided by the government to anyone who bothered to visit. They were equipped with just a few Paracetamol tablets, and some dubious looking coloured tablets which I discovered were multivitamins which worked well as placebos. There were a few red-coloured cough syrups, and a lot of Voveran injections that took care of most pain-related emergencies. The basic primary health centres took care of most of the health emergencies and very few had to visit tertiary care hospitals. The lifesaver in our centre was the peon-cum-guard, Ram Saran. He doubled as our medical adviser. Having dealt with endless 'fresh off the boat' doctors, he was well-versed with our ignorant situation. He knew that we knew nothing about any medicines or any diagnosis. In short, he knew we were a long way off from being doctors. As soon as a patient entered, he would call out loudly, "Doctor, an appendicitis patient is here." As we scrambled to our feet rubbing our eyes, he would smile and hand the Voveran injection to one of us. He would wrap a few multivitamin capsules for the patient to take home. As all doctors in the world know, renal colic, gall bladder colic, appendicitis emergencies, vomiting, babies crying incessantly, all have a propensity to occur in the middle of the night. I think that humanity has colluded against doctors to prevent them from having a full night's sleep.

The next night, it would be a loud, "Renal stone, Doctor." Arising from our slumber in the small side rooms (meant for doctors on night duty), one of us would trudge wearily to the emergency room, rubbing her eyes. Ram Saran would be ready with an ampule of Voveran injection to allay the patients' symptoms and our fear of diagnosing. It didn't seem fair to be woken up at night to shove a Voveran injection into someone's backside, since we were perpetually weary from endless cycling and chatting during the day.

The only consolation was that we never had to rack our

brains about a diagnosis or line of treatment since Ram Saran knew everything. His tremendous knowledge did not make him insufferable. Always respectful, he addressed us as Doctor saheb with the right degree of deference, appropriate for the difference in his and our positions. After all, we were doctors!

With Ram Saran in our lives, our rural posting felt like a big holiday. We cooked, cycled and chatted away until the wee hours and, of course, we took many pictures. Learning to be a doctor was the last thing that crossed our minds.

As I stood with Father on the farmland, with Baburam gazing at me as if I had descended from the heavens just to treat him, I felt so alone. I missed Ram Saran, the peon. He would have told me the diagnosis discreetly as he always did. Hearing Father declare me as a new-found, magical doctor with his unimaginable flair and pride, made me recoil with diffidence. The more assuredness Father displayed in my skills, the more doubts I had of them.

As the story goes, Baburam had been suffering from fever for over a month and had been visiting some village quacks for treatment.

"Check his pulse," Father prodded me gently as he saw me at a loss for actions or words.

Of course, I thought. Everyone except me seemed to know what had to be done.

I looked intently at Baburam's hand. I would and should have looked at the pulse, but the thought of holding that sweaty, calloused hand made me cringe and I looked away from it.

"There is no need," I stated with as much authority and composure as I could muster, for there was no way I was going to touch that sweaty, smelly hand.

I am better than this, my heart cried every moment.

I pretended to be in deep thought about the diagnosis and looked beyond Baburam at the new grass. It works, the thinking act. Patients respect the fact that the doctor thought deeply before declaring a diagnosis.

"Get a chest X-ray and a typhoid test," I said after an appropriate, thoughtful interval, tilting my chin up a bit to reflect authority as I would in Kalawati Saran Hospital.

Baburam and Father glared at me in disbelief, their eyes wide, as if I had told Baburam to recite Shakespeare.

"No, no, that is not possible," said Father quickly. "You just give him some tablets. I am sure you can diagnose him just like that."

I stared at Father exasperated, as one would at an unreasonable child. Little did I know that diagnosing 'just like that' would become the magic phrase forever and for a lifetime. Battling to decide my next step, I could see Baburam standing in his 'dirty from working at the farm' loincloth with his gaze plastered on my face, not leaving it for a moment lest I disappear. He waited for me to pull out some magic potion or wave a wand over his head. However, when no magic wand emerged from my bag, I could see he looked a tad disappointed but continued with his relentless gaping. This was the first time I had diagnosed anyone with prolonged fever without a chest X-ray or a blood test.

Never again! I told myself. I was used to having a whole back-up of laboratories and seniors that I could fall back on. At that moment, I stood wretched under the blazing May sun and missed having a team.

Baburam and Father continued their unfettered and

highly expectant appraisal of my face as I whittled down the long list of causes of fever in my mind. The list of differential diagnosis of fevers was one of the questions in the final year examinations, hence, was fresh in my mind. Typhoid seemed the most plausible cause, so most definitely it was that. I took a confident chance, as I couldn't afford to appear shaky with the two men peering into my face, "I think it's Typhoid," I said resolutely and rattled off some medicines for Typhoid. No one seemed to have any paper, so the names of the medicines flew off into the gentle breeze. I repeated, a bit slowly this time. Father cut me short with, "There is no chemist here, so you give me the list in the car." He was happy to obtain them the next day and I conveniently let him bask in his enthusiasm.

The following morning, Father had procured the medicines that I had asked for and waited eagerly to drive me to the farm. By some stroke of heavenly luck, Baburam was as fit as a fiddle within three to four days. If he had not returned to work in three days with his toothy smile, my life would have taken me to a big London hospital. Baburam had become the dice in this providential game. On the fourth day, he rounded up five more people from his village—people who had the same fever, he said. And yes, I had to diagnose them 'just like that'. To my utter surprise, all of them became fitter than before. I had never seen anyone look so fit in four days. Nature was also colluding against me in the downgrading of my life and career. More drives happened in the following days. In fact, the drives to the farm became a daily affair as more farm workers became fitter and better. Strangely, I found myself looking forward to going to the farm. Maybe it was the novelty of the farm or maybe it was the bright welcome I received from Baburam and his team of new men every day.

A week later, Mother accompanied us in the car. It was highly unusual for her to be going to the farm so I wondered why. My highly-developed, educated sense told me that it wasn't important. That assumption was a big mistake! How could I have known that this was going to be a life changing day for me!

As I sat in the car with her, my mind pulled out abstractions from her life.

Mother was the gentlest and most silent person I can remember. Being married myself for many years, I cannot understand how I never heard her arguing with Father. Never did I ever hear a word of disagreement or discord in our home. She just accepted. She accepted all his anxious moments, his fears, his involvement with the farm, his angry moments and his large-heartedness with the same silent equanimity. At twenty-five, full of my own views, the enormity of her silence was incomprehensible. I thought that her silence was just part of her personality and probably she had nothing to say. Back then, the importance of silence that occurs within a marriage was lost on me. As I grew older and had discords, big and small with my husband, I tried to follow her example, but it was impossible not to dissent and to prove my convictions loud and clear. In my sixties, my respect for her has grown because I understand that she was not without a voice or an opinion. Her silence had a certain strength which had to be admired because it kept the family sane and together.

How did she manage to keep her balance with a husband and four children? How did she manage to be silent when she had so much to say?

Never once did she question my expenses, my friends or

my outings with boys. How did she keep her calm when I lied to her in my teenage enthusiasm? I always wonder if she ever grieved when I made blunders. Did she suffer from guilt pangs and question herself where she had gone wrong as a mother? It surely must have been an agony to hold back and let me wander the dark alleys of adolescence. How did she trust me unquestionably and unconditionally? I have tried to grant my daughter the same trust and unconditional faith. In my overprotectiveness, I know I fall short compared to her.

Why was she going to the farm? Maybe she was going to see the progress of the farm. Maybe she wanted to see the party lawns or maybe she liked potholed roads; maybe she was bored that day or maybe she wanted to go for a drive with me, her dear daughter. My mind cavorted with various theories as I sat quietly. For everyone else too, it was a quiet drive. As the farm came into sight, I saw a huge blue board on the wall of the guard room, just outside the farm gate. I hadn't seen it before on my earlier visits. It was so big that it pygmied everything else around. It took me a while to register that it had my name printed on it in the largest and boldest letters—DR BALESH JINDAL.

I cringed in distaste and said, "Oh it's so big!" My words fell on deaf ears, literally. No one looked at me as father and mother were both busy admiring the big board and smiling happily. They looked at each other and smiled some more. I stared at the sign in dismay and could not stand it, so I looked away without a word. No one was listening anyway.

"It is just perfect," Father exclaimed as he beamed at Mother for her sanction. She smiled in approval and turned to look back at me in the backseat. She always agreed with Father so there was no point in expecting any support from her. I refused to meet her eyes and pretended to stare out of the window to show my displeasure. Stealing another look at the board, I winced in embarrassment and looked away again. My name in the big, bold letters made me feel proportionally small. The size of the letters outsized the board of Kalawati Saran Hospital too, and it proclaimed loud and clear that here I was, someone with no options in life, someone who needed a big signboard to feel important. Glowering at Father, I saw that he was unfazed in his enthusiasm. I tried to unravel his intent. What did the board mean? Maybe he just wanted to see his daughter's name on a board, or maybe he just liked big boards. He knew I was leaving for London, then what was that gigantic board doing on that wall?

As we alighted from the car, Father fell in step with me and he must have noticed my gloom and quiet. He moved near me gently and said quietly, "Rest assured, this is just a stopgap arrangement and you are free to plan what to do in life." An undue stress on free, I sensed, perhaps a euphemism for 'twiddling your thumbs'. His warm brown eyes looked at me and he added in a resigned tone, "You can leave anytime."

I knew there was nothing left to argue after this subtle and final statement.

How much time the young waste in the pigmented illusions of their vaingloriousness and self-aggrandisation, so preoccupied by the flippant arrogance of their youth and unfounded sureness! I know this because if I had shared and comprehended Father's forevision of this glorious practice in 1983, I would have embraced the opportunity with hope and gratitude instead of sorrow.

I stood at the farm dejected and depleted, joyless in the

belief that I was being pushed into a doomed future. This foreboding of darkness and desolation marred many years that followed. My youthful presumptions and conditioned ideas of success stripped me of all happiness and content that I could have enjoyed with the success of my clinic. For decades I continued to rue my luck and wallowed in the dreariness of my situation. All forms of self-respect, confidence and pride eluded me due to the constricted span of my comprehension. I wish I had enjoyed the glorious journey with an open mind—a regret I had rather late in life,

When we entered the small clinic, Baburam had just finished lighting a small holy fire for a 'havan' to initiate me on the path of charity. A priest in pristine white clothes prepared to start the havan. He mumbled some mantras and watched us as we found our places on the jute durries spread around the fire. As soon as Baburam saw me, he rushed to touch my feet. I recoiled, but the touching of the feet became the norm in the days and times to come.

"This is for good luck and good omen," Father said with affection as he gestured towards the smoky offering, expecting me to sit beside him. Like a sacrificial lamb, I crossed my legs and sat in front of the holy fire. Mother, too, crossed her legs and sat close to me, her hand on mine, protectively. The bright yellow marigold flowers from the farm lay scattered around the fire. They looked pretty, I noted grudgingly. The morning sun flooded the room with rays that seemed to drench everyone in a warm way.

I looked around as two women wearing long cotton skirts entered the room and sat close to each other on one of the five wooden benches that were laid around the room, next to the wall. Their faces were half veiled with a bright cotton cloth revealing only bright, inquisitive eyes. On the heels of the two women, a man entered and on seeing the holy fire and the havan that was underway, he folded his hands, closed his eyes and bowed towards the flames in obeisance and then sat on one of the waiting benches. Another man entered shortly after with a kid in his arms. The child appeared to be wheezing. I was busy glancing between the flames and this influx of strange people. I knew that the situation was not in my control as I could not comprehend the larger picture. I kept trying to decipher the events in my head but drew a blank.

It was obvious that I was missing an important link. The holy fire and the big board were two links that seemed suspicious.

By the time the ceremony finished, all four benches were filled with an assorted collection of people, their eyes closed as they swayed in rhythm with the *mantras* being recited by the priest. They all looked at peace with themselves and their surroundings. It seemed I was the only one who was not at peace that morning. There must have been about twenty people I counted, and wondered as to why they were sitting there. Maybe they had come for the sweets, as I had seen some sweet boxes stacked on a table. Of course, they had come for the sweets! I prided myself for my innate understanding of situations. I could feel that there was an air of deep reverence that filled the room along with the sunlight. That itself was another suspicious link. It felt like I had been projected into a hallowed environment in one fell swoop. Everyone sat with eyes closed, folded hands in their laps and heads bowed low.

Father bent towards me and said quietly, "Look at the respect these people have for you." Little does he know, I thought cryptically, as I was certain that the respect was for him as he was the landowner. His inability to see this glaring fact was understandable, as he hadn't read the books that I had and didn't have my insight. I was more aware and well-read and was proud of my knowledge and maturity even though he was an astute businessman.

As the *havan* came to an end and the priest stood up and dusted his white dhoti, Baburam hurtled himself towards the sweets boxes and started to distribute them as *prasad.* The people on the benches took their boxes but didn't walk out as I thought they would. I was surprised as they all sat back again on the benches. Somewhere I was missing something! It was very baffling even to a person as logical as me. I decided not to tire myself over some inconsequential happenings and started to walk out to sit in the car that would take me home. That is when Father caught up with me from behind, smiled and gestured towards the patients "This is your practice. They are your patients. You are free to take it or leave it."

What was I thinking? How could I have missed all the signs? It dawned on me that all the strangers who had filled the benches were patients. They had come to me with their ailments expecting miracles. I considered feigning a headache and telling Father that I felt sick or I could lie to him and say that I had made other plans and leave, but I did nothing of that sort. I quietly walked back to the room with the benches and the people on them. They were no longer people. They were patients. I glanced around to gather my bearings and assess the surroundings. I knew I was defeated.

My patients! Suddenly I was related to them in a doctor-patient relationship.

How could I have misread the situation so wrong? Was I tricked into the practice? No! Not at all. Father said over and again, "You can take it or leave it." It was my choice. Even on the first day, I could have walked out and not treated those people sitting on the benches. I know that somewhere the desire to help these villagers was pushing me forward for this practice.

Baburam became my undesignated compounder for the day as he was eager to help and I didn't have anyone else. He herded one patient at a time and led them out when I had finished with them.

This was officially the first day at my clinic. I was twenty-five.

As I gathered my wits around me, I saw that the clinic had two rooms. The outside one was obviously a large waiting room. It had large windows and the sun spilled in with unexpected fervour as if enjoying my discomfiture. This was the room where everyone had sat for the puja. The inside room was my consultancy room. It was tiny by hospital standards. There was a table, an office chair for me and just enough space to move around. A small wooden stool sat near my table for the patients to sit on, right next to me. Luckily, I had carried my beloved stethoscope and blood pressure apparatus from my Kalawati days in a bag, in expectation of examining two or three of Baburam's men.

Once settled in my new workspace, I began examining the patients.

The child who had been wheezing in the outside room during the prayers had to be the first one for I could hear his wheezing and it had become faster and louder. After examining him I wrote bronchodilators for him and made notes of all the medicines that had to be bought for the next day as now I knew that these people had no access to a chemist. The child clearly needed his medicines today as he was wheezing badly. Tomorrow might be too late and he could not be allowed to go home. The most obvious action was to take him in the car with us and drop him at the nearest chemist. By doing this, I would be defeating my purpose of protesting against the clinic. Helping this patient could be certainly misconstrued as an assent from my side. Saving the child took precedence over my protest. I don't remember how I justified this action to my irate self. I found myself telling the father of the wheezing child to wait for me as the rest of the patients had to be seen.

"My knees ache so much," said the old lady in the white skirt.

"How many days?"

"Many years, five years...maybe six."

"Why didn't you show earlier?" It was an irrelevant question, I realised the moment it left my mouth. Obviously there were no doctors in these villages.

Strangely, I started to feel bad for them. No, no, don't, I warned myself.

I had a clear view of the waiting room from my big chair in the consultation room. Then a wrinkled old woman walked in. She probably had a wrinkle for every year of her age, just like tree trunks. There was a vague vulnerability in her wrinkledness as she walked in quietly towards the stool. She pulled at her scarlet dupatta that was flung across her neck to wipe a small, inadvertent tear. When she saw me looking at her, the tears turned to a faint, happy smile. My gaze went to her crooked teeth. It had to, for they shone bright in her face. They were crooked alright but seemed more agreeable than crooked teeth could ever be. As she limped in with an irregular gait, I could see that she could not straighten her back. She sat and rested her arm on her long walking stick that looked like a thick pole of the 'pole vault' variety. She just sat there and looked at me, without a word, with wondrous eyes. She moved near my table and reached out for my hand. She cupped it with hers and tried to show me where her back hurt. Under the guidance of her hand, my hand slid down her back just below the rib cage. She held on to my hand firmly and guided it lower and lower, till it reached the lower lumbar region. I touched it peremptorily just to make her happy. The moment my hand reached the correct destination, she smiled and let go of it. She put her hand gently on my head as a gesture of blessing. "I will get alright now with your touch. It's good you came here beta, you are God." She smiled and turned to walk away.

"Wait, Amma, do take some medicine for the pain," I mumbled, unsure of the right words. Two other women had been looking intently at the whole examination. "She will get okay by your touch," said the one in the yellow dupatta and nodded her head.

"She just wanted you to touch her with your magic," smiled another wearing a bead necklace, a bit loudly as she sat waiting for her turn. "We can't believe that a real doctor has come to treat us," she said in quiet veneration. "Our *kismet* will change now."

"Why did she have tears in her eyes?" I asked her.

"They were tears of disbelief and happiness at seeing you."

This was just the first day.

To say I was moved would be understating the fact that I was shaken.

It was understood that I was important for myself and my family, but it was a new experience that I could be so important and mean so much to people who were strangers. This was a new realisation!

I set about examining the rest of the people. The picture of the old woman who had walked away flashed before me constantly even as I busied myself with the waiting crowd. Some of the people had backaches and a bit of pain in the knees and all they needed were painkillers, anti-inflammatory tablets and plenty of calcium. It was certain that they had conjured up the ailments just to have a look at me, the new doctor. An old man lumbered into my room, breathless. At first glance, his eyes were red. Bloodshot! He was unmistakably a farmer as his face wore a farmer's wrinkles and ruddiness as deep as furrows in a field. I found these unapologetic furrows very quaint. He walked over to the small stool and sat beside me. I studied his face and surmised that he wasn't as old as he looked. Looking at his eyes carefully it was apparent that the redness wasn't due to an infection, an inner sense told me. I checked his blood pressure and was taken aback at the results—190/110 mm hg. When I measured it again it showed the same reading.

"I have to start medicines for hypertension." He stared at me with distrust and doubt. Doubts about my knowledge, experience and qualifications clouded his furrowed face because I was new. "You are new here," he said patronisingly, in response to my diagnosis that he presumed stemmed from my scant knowledge of medicine.

"It's just gas and acidity. I never take medicine for anything.

Besides, my old doctor in the village just gives me syrup for gas." He got up to leave, but I knew that if he went home unconvinced, word would get around and everyone else would lose faith in me. Looking at him squarely in the face I said, "This much blood pressure is not good. If you don't want any medicine for the blood pressure, I will not put you on any medication today." He seemed to relent at this option of no medication. Picking up the encouraging cue, I advised him bed rest, a salt restricted diet, and gave him a syrup for gas. An important lesson I learnt on my first day was to sense what the patient wanted and to give it to them without much ado, especially if it was as harmless as an antacid.

"Let me put you under observation." It was like putting my foot in the door hoping to open it later. He promised to come daily to get his blood pressure measured and it was obvious that I had won a tiny battle, which was enough for my first day.

A couple of other patients had minor coughs and colds. Fortunately, there wasn't anything too serious on my first day at the clinic. I heaved a sigh of relief when the day came to an end. While making my way to the car, I saw the man with the wheezing child sitting on his haunches near the car. Father gestured to him to get in. Once in the car, Father was a sight to be seen. He kept looking over his shoulder at my board, back at me and then at Mother. His dream had come true.

The patient sat in the back next to me. He was sweaty and smelly. Strangely it did not bother me because the child had to be saved. He sat still and quietly in the back seat till we dropped him in front of the first chemist shop that we saw. "Thank you for making a clinic in Kapashera," he said to me as he walked into the shop.

I saw a joyful achievement on my father's face as he drove home.

"You can go to England or stay here," he said once again and I knew he meant it. Had I been less grumpy that summer day and had shared the happiness he felt at seeing the people who sat around the holy fire, his joy would have been complete. The *havan,* the priest, the many people who turned out to be patients and the guard room with the huge board had overwhelmed me and I knew I was incapable of emoting anymore that day.

The drive home was steeped in my father's unreserved jubilation, while I sat sullen, sulky and silent. Silence was the only way to protest against the clinic. I lost track of the plans he was chalking out for me as we drove back home, for I was still reeling from the turn of events that day. Catching random snippets from his conversation I gathered that he planned to make a full-fledged hospital for me. I was comforted by the fact that we would be going to London anyway so refuting his ideas in the car would serve no purpose. I remained quiet as it was pointless being pettish and truncating his joy. Mother listened to him as always, spellbound and nodding her head at all his grand plans. We continued our journey back home. After a long while on the bumpy road, the car screeched to a stop and I was home.

"By next year you will have your own hospital," my father said with a heightened elation, his face glowing, as the car stopped in front of my new marital home. I remained quiet, a bit exhausted with all the strategising and resisting all morning. The following morning, Father was ready in the car and we headed for the clinic once again.

In the winter of 1983, my husband returned from his stint in England. He came back with new dreams in his eyes—dreams of going back to England. I was eager to accompany him to this faraway land of fairytales, where I could be the best paediatrician ever. Soon Kapashera would be behind us. Like most good things in life, that did not happen. England fell off the horizon for my husband too, due to certain reasons. He had to remain in India, which disturbed and disappointed him for a while. Later he got a good appointment in a big tertiary care hospital where he could operate and teach. I resigned myself to the existence of the clinic, which was to become a permanent reality for me.

CHAPTER TWO

The Uncertain Doctor

"Respond to adversity, real or imagined, not with self-pity or hand wringing, but simply by starting over."
Eric Weiner, *The Socrates Express*

THERE WERE NO chemists in any of the surrounding villages, so obtaining the simplest of medicines became an uphill battle for me and the patients. Procuring medicines in wholesale and storing them in the clinic became integral to my practice. The concept of writing down a prescription was unheard of and simply not practical, which I learnt the hard way. If I ever wrote anything on my new letterheads, that patient would invariably return a month or two later and say, "I haven't got well. Your medicines did not help one bit."

"Did you take them regularly?" I asked Ram Lal, a patient with an infected, ingrown toenail.

"No, I did not buy them. I could not find these anywhere," he said as he thrust my crumpled prescription towards me.

"So, how would you get well?" I asked, veiling my frustration.

"Well, I tried a few shops. I went all over," he said, exasperated with my questions.

I knew he must have tried.

"Did you go to a chemist shop?"

"No, I went to the big shop—the one that has everything from shoes to toys and shirts." He winced in pain. Obviously, he had gone to a general store and I could see that his toenail was swollen, red and badly infected causing him severe pain and discomfort.

"Why didn't you come earlier?" I said although I knew it was a silly question.

"I could have got the medicines for you."

"I had sowing to do in my field for it's time to sow the wheat," he explained patiently even as his desperation to get back to his sowing was obvious from his hurried speech. So that was it. I needed to have my own pharmacy and dispensing solutions which was another step down into the steep well that I was already in. The thought of being a consultant flew out of the window. A rural clinic with a general practice instead of a specialist one, and if I started dispensing, I would be sinking deeper into a pit of failure but it had to be done.

I solved the problem of availability of medicines by making a list of all essential medical supplies. Within a week, I was in business. Father procured the complete list of equipment and medicines I had written in longhand. A thermometer, a weighing machine, a torch, a letter pad, a few antibiotics, painkillers, a stainless-steel steriliser, a pestle and mortar, paper packets for dispensing medicines and plastic bottles for mixtures and syrups for small kids. Tetanus vials, most of the common vaccines, some shots for epilepsy, a nebuliser for asthmatic kids and Voveran vials for renal and gallbladder colics were all stocked. Wasn't I glad to have obtained this miracle injection Voveran! It cured the pain caused by stones, renal, gallbladder and all others. After all, the colics did constitute the commonest emergencies!

Gradually, I set out to stock my clinic with more medicines and continued to add, as my repertoire of illnesses and patients grew. Generic drugs were one-fourth of the price of branded drugs and were as effective so I went for them, warily at first but confidently later. This reduced the cost of treatment for almost all infections. By stocking the best antibiotics, I received the most optimum response in the shortest time possible and, believe it or not, the much-maligned generic drugs offered me excellent results for nearly four decades. I used them by default as they were considerably cheaper and I wasn't aware of their downmarket reputation. Later, during group discussions with colleagues, I learnt that it was not okay to use these as they were not considered efficient compared to the more expensive branded drugs. It was better to keep my secret to myself and I continued to use them happily. As the years went by, I learnt more about pricing, profitability and cost-effectiveness, and steadily I acquired generic drugs from wholesalers and manufacturers directly.

My letterheads came a week later and it was heady to see my name with Lady Hardinge and Kalawati Saran inscribed at the top. The patients started to come in, some just to have a look at the new doctor, others to actually receive free advice on some chronic illness. For a long time, I felt like I was the one being tested and examined.

If I were to treat the patients with any scientific evidence, having my own blood testing facilities seemed imperative. There were no laboratories for even basic blood tests anywhere in the area. Initially, I worked on presumptions, guess work and, of course, hunches. Typhoid, jaundice, malaria, pleuritis, ascitis, anaemia, septicaemia, diabetes and the whole gamut of infections were all diagnosed by purposeful auscultation with my Litman stethoscope, deep percussion taught by the fussy professor of medicine Dr Hiranandani, and most importantly keen observation. A good history became invaluable to diagnosing. Even as I took detailed history I knew that it was not a long-term solution. Blood investigations are the backbone of any medical practice. A microscope, a centrifuge, a few test tubes, pipettes, and testing solutions made their way to my shelves. Every afternoon, once the last patient left, would see me doing haemoglobin and blood sugar, typhoid, blood group, and urine infections. Blood investigations remained a small part of the diagnosis paraphernalia as I relied more on my senses. With the internet, things have changed. Patients now rely more on the laboratory reports than on the doctor and most of them come armed, at first consultation, with possible diagnosis of their ailments downloaded from Google.

The daily drives with Father grew on me as he drove me to the clinic every single morning. His pride and enthusiasm for the clinic never showed the slightest signs of waning. I had never interacted with him so much before the birth of the clinic, living in the hostel for five years and being immersed in memorising thick and intensive books and being busy with endless night duties, I had no time to notice people called parents. Long drives to the farm meant long, unhurried conversations. To learn how important it was to him that I practise medicine in a place where there were no facilities available, I found myself understanding his dream. He had bought the farm partly because of this, he admitted on one drive.

The number of patients mushroomed and came mostly from the surrounding villages of Kapashera, Samalkha and Bijwasan. Some travelled from distant villages such as Dhulsiras, Bamnoli, Daulatpur, Chawla, Nangal Devat, Palam and Rajokri. Furthermore, there were a lot of them from Vasant Kunj, an extensive habitation a few kilometres away. Patients even commuted from faraway places such as Sikanderpur, Badshahpur, Kanganheri, Najafgarh and Sultanpur. Rewari was a few hours by road and several of them came from there. I would look in disbelief when some patients informed me of their five-hour commute to reach my clinic. The patients from Kapashera and Rajokri lived close enough to walk to my clinic and would arrive at nine or earlier and wait patiently on the pavement outside for my car to whizz to a stop. The most poignant thing was that some of them from far-off villages would hitch rides in a tractor or a random interstate bus and reach my clinic in the early hours and wait patiently for me.

There was an old neem tree just outside the clinic. That became my parking space. Groups of patients would sit comfortably under the neem tree or perched on their haunches on the sidewalk on most mornings waiting for the shutters of the clinic to open. Most of the men would be puffing at their beedis happily. The affluent ones would be gurgling away on a hookah, their big turbans sitting regally on their grey hair, as that was a luxury only a few could afford. The assortment of these patients kept my parking space free of other vehicles. Other vehicles comprised bullock carts loaded with sacks of wheat to be taken to the wholesale mandi or fodder for their cows, tractors, lone cows, goats, hand-pulled rickshaws, bicycles and a random motorcycle. At times some lone woman would get her donkey to the clinic and tie the animal to the electric pole while she finished her business with me.

As soon as I got out of the car, people would file into the clinic just on my heels and sit patiently on the wooden benches waiting to be called in. I felt guilty for making them wait even though their faces displayed no signs of accusation or grouch.

In this part of the world all the daily chores were guided by the sun. It was natural since no one owned a watch. Somehow their timing was perfect. Some would say, "Please call me out of turn as I have a long way to go. I want to reach home before the sun sets."

It was easy to oblige these special requests as the waiting patients did not seem to mind if anyone was called out of turn. It was amazing to see their patience and fortitude as these illiterate people were a far cry from the educated circle of people that I was familiar with. They were an accommodative lot, ready to give up their position in the queue without a fuss.

If asked when they had eaten their breakfast, the answer would be "Just after sunrise."

"When did you get the pain in your stomach?"

"Just before I milked my cows," which was always at four in the evening for most homes. Knowing the sunrise and sunset timings, and timing for milking, feeding and bathing the cows was essential and went a long way in saving time to elicit history. In fact, I stopped wearing a watch to see if I could sense the time of day from the movement of the sun across the sky. Good knowledge of the distances of the neighbouring villages came in handy as I would dispense extra medicines to them to reduce the number of visits and travel costs. Patients from a village further away received special attention and a place higher up in the queue. I called them before others so they could reach home before dark.

The water coolers in the clinic whirred constantly and the waiting room became a cool haven, away from the scorching summer sun. Some old men and women sat in the coolness to keep out the midday sun as they waited for their turn. Maybe their visit was for some cool air and cold water or to get some respite from their daily lives. In the eighties, people had no access to coolers, cold water or even toilets. They would look wondrously at the toilet and loved to hear the sound of the water rattling down the flush. Some came as one would to a club, hoping for some camaraderie and conversations. Finding a man or woman eager to make small talk and laugh with was not difficult as the waiting room had many contenders for that. I ensured a chilled drinking water supply and trained my staff of two village girls to offer cold water from the fridge to all the patients. They had to address the patients with the appropriate salutations. I was particular about these behaviours when I trained these simple girls. They were good learners as they were middle school dropouts and belonged to the villages so were one of them. Being dropouts they wanted to prove themselves and tried hard. The moment I heard a hint of irritation or peevishness in the girls' tone, they were reprimanded.

"Treat the patients as you would treat your guests," I taught them.

Patients started to flock to the clinic for non-existent ailments. I knew they had come for some reassuring words from me. Some older women would come with a supposed pain in their little finger or an apparent ball of gas rolling in their stomach. Their metaphors and similes were ingenuous and confounded me at first. Later, I learnt to decipher their lingo. They were village folks, so their diseases came with rustic descriptions. These weren't mentioned in any of the medical books that I had read.

"My head is churning like a ball of butter!" This was a bit dicey as it could be dizziness due to vertigo or purely psychosomatic.

"My leg hurts as if a cow had hit me." Of course, this meant it was severe in intensity and had to be muscular spasm or osteoarthritis.

"I had a lot of makki roti (corn) last night, and my stomach feels like a balloon." The obvious interpretation was gastritis.

"My skin is crawling with tiny worms; I can't sleep." This was scabies, for sure.

"My body is aching as if I was beaten by ten men." I knew this one, I thought gleefully. Post fever myalgia!

There were a lot of casualties caused by cows and buffalos, of varying degrees of grievousness. During milking the cow, it was not uncommon for the cow to act up and deliver a fine kick to the person sitting under. Since these were randomly inflicted they were varied and difficult to diagnose.

If someone's daughter-in-law visited me for pain in the abdomen, which seemed to have no origin and did not fit into any cause, I knew her problem could be related to back-breaking cattle work. A daughter's looming marriage, an aggressive son or a violent and alcoholic husband were all causes of diseases that were unrelated to any physical causes. It took a few years for me to recognise these symptoms and not go in for a battery of investigations. The clinic became a happy place to come to.

'The patient is, so we are,' was my motto.

In November 1985, my husband and I were blessed with a beautiful baby boy. I took a paltry ten days' maternity leave from the clinic. Why did I do that? I do not know? Being away from the practice for ten days made me realise that it had made inroads into my psyche and had become an inseparable part of me. It just wasn't any clinic; it was 'my clinic'.

Father stood in for me for those ten days and handed out the medicines to my patients. He asked me details on the phone and I guided my staff to wrap up the correct doses for the poor villagers. They were rickshaw-pullers, labourers, masons and factory workers. He attended to them because he did not want anyone to go back without medicine. Father ran one of the leading paper industries of the country and his cars were the talk of the town. His fancy red Sedan, probably the first in the city, whizzed fast on Delhi roads. Yet, he stood in my clinic, in his loose kurta-pyjama, handing out medicines to poor labourers and daily wagers. "They come from far away and should not go back without medicine," he kept repeating.

That was his dedication and drive!

How could I leave?

Even as I immersed myself in the rural clinic, my heart yearned for my life that was.

It was the year 1972 and Father's business started growing by leaps and bounds; and I developed a natural fondness for the finer things of life such as modern clothes, going for coffee outings, watching movies and dancing in the new clubs. Sipping champagne at a romantic garden party and delicately balancing the stem of the exquisite goblet within the soft clasp of my fingers was one of the most preferred activities for me.

There were no curfews at night and no limit on my spending, drinking and whatever restrictions parents set in those days for their children, especially girls. Father ensured that I had the latest dresses to be the star of every gathering, and to repeat any dress for parties that I attended was sacrilege. Even at a young age, I could fathom that good grades were directly proportional to Father's generosity. Somehow, it so happened that good grades were not challenging to come by. It was an exhilarating existence. With my proven sane judgement and judicious thinking, Father trusted me to a fault. My three brothers had many rules imposed upon them for Father did not trust their judgement as he did mine. Every decision I took, my mind always went to Father and I would ask myself, 'Will this make him proud?'

This one lone question sustained me safely through life.

My lifestyle would surely be termed decadent by most. What else would a seventeen-year-old youngster need?

I need to mention all these privileges I had because the next forty years of my life were filled with irony and paradoxes of the highest order. It was the experience and memory of this affluent lifestyle that helped me to overcome squalor, disdain and hardships of a life that was to be.

Even while I was in school, Father had already set his sights on Lady Hardinge Medical College and planned that his daughter would drive to that prestigious institution in her beautiful new car. It was the year 1976.

Just a handful of people owned cars in Delhi at that time. The parking lot had rows of black motorcycles, which were owned by the 'wanting to appear sexy' young doctors. Another row was allocated for scooters, which were owned by the safety conscious senior professors. It had just one shiny green and white Fiat that stood out for its sheer beauty—that was my car. I did not realise the effect it had on the entire college. I was judged, shunned, envied by most and revered by a few.

A good friend Sheema and I would bunk classes and the boring afternoon tutorials and drive down to the IIT campus. Everyone knew it had the best guys. We hoped that if we just loitered on the road inside the campus we could find a respectable boyfriend. This activity continued for the entire second and third years. Then the practical ward rounds started which made me feel like a real doctor and the priorities changed, from hunting for a respectable boyfriend in IIT to learning to become a good doctor.

From being a fashion leader and an ambitious person, a rural clinic was a big step down in life. It was a free fall, free for all to see as I lost my coveted pedestal. I went about the daily disheartening drives down NH8 to my small clinic. I knew that the old cloak of privilege that had ensconced me had been ripped away for it was redundant in Kapashera. There would be no England, no paediatrics, no pencil skirts and no romantic parties.

It didn't help that my colleagues and friends held me in disregard and disinterest due to my lack of specialisation and for running an insubstantial rural clinic. I shirked all friends and colleagues as much as they did me. This was enough cause for my longanimity. The dreams of going to the UK and of becoming the best paediatrician ever had quietly funnelled their way into the darkness of the reality of the clinic.

Life flowed along in my feigned nonchalance in what my colleagues were achieving on the professional front. The desolation and disgust of the initial years changed to a silent resentment and then to a resigned acceptance.

The assumption that I had accepted an easy life over anything challenging haunted me. Disappointment of quashed ambitions and a botched up career remained for decades. It was not easy because it had taken my entire girlhood to nurture and incubate them. One can't toss away things of value in a flash. It hurt like hell! It did!

It was the year 2014 that became the year of enlightenment. Like a flash it hit me, and I realised that what I had was indeed precious and worthy. A truth that dawned on me extremely late in life. I learnt that the clinic was not a degradation. I just needed a wider vision to look at my situation through a different lens—a vision that got buried with my 'highly educated and learned sense'. As Thoreau has said, 'From the right point of view, every storm and every drop in it is a rainbow'. So it was in 2014 that I started to respect myself once again.

I learnt that passion was not akin to happiness.

Passions can be changed; so can ambitions. It's the environmental circumstances that guide passion and ambition. To chase personal targets may not lead to a fulfilled life; one has to retarget. Even though the clinic was not my idea of an ideal practice, I pursued it, redesigning my path as I went along. That became my unlearning and my absolution.

I survived repeating words of wisdom to myself like, "If one finds oneself against the tide, swim with grace and dignity."

When did the patients merge with my own priorities and psyche and became one entity? Well, I do not know. The patients amalgamated with my identity because I did not compartmentalise life enough as most people do. I let the patients occupy all the compartments of my mind and heart till they mushroomed into a spate that drowned everything. There was place for very little else.

I do believe in destiny. I firmly believe that mine had been carved out for me since time immemorial. The thousands of people who thronged my clinic, the waiting room that ran out of space and the patients that waited on the pavement outside, the lengthening waiting time for a patient to see me, these were signs that my presence in Kapashera was meant to be.

It was preordained.

How could I leave?

How could I disappoint the hundreds and thousands of people who needed a doctor, and most importantly, how could I let Father down?

How could I shatter Father's dreams?

And so, I stayed.

Father continued to drive me to the clinic every day. In the eighties and nineties, the words charity and compassion were not an entity. We just did what we could and there was no social media to post our goodness on a daily basis. I just flowed with the tide and did my best, hoping that my best was good enough.

I was humbled by Father's pleasure at seeing these people come from far and wide. He would pop in around mid-afternoon with a bottle of cold buttermilk for me. He lingered around in the clinic with joy exuding from his face, looking at the patients, looking at me examining them and smiling when they smiled. He never tried to mask his pride. I had never seen him so happy and this happiness was enough for me to know that I was doing the right thing.

"Never turn a patient away for want of money or time," he would repeat slowly. His words ring clear in my mind even today.

How could I leave?

One winter afternoon, the mustard fields were in full bloom. They dazzled the eyes as the sun shone on their yellowness. The farm was coming along well; the flower beds were blooming and spring was on its way. Father drove as we made our way home. He talked about his earlier days and how hard he had worked to reach where he was now. He spoke about the first car he had bought which was a second-hand Morris, and he discussed the progress of the farm.

That was the last day he drove me to the clinic.

He met with a road accident that very afternoon which left me completely shattered. It was not just an accident. The foundations of our existence crumbled and threatened to destroy everything we held dear. Father was the centre of many businesses—the factories, the offices, the farm and hundreds of workers all lost a father that day.

I took it upon myself to console Mother who was inconsolable and devastated. She could barely hold herself—so silent was the arrival of death, so loud the effect! Sudden and fatal! It was like a storm that flattened everything in sight.

There were many old relatives who descended on us. People we hadn't seen for years now moved around the house as if they lived there. Seeing an opportunity, everyone wanted to advise. I had to protect Mother from the Indian custom of breaking her glass bangles and removing her sindoor and the red bindi that she wore. These were sacred signs of a married woman.

I stood by her side and did not let any of the toxic relatives near her. Some women insisted that she remove her bangles. Seeing my sharp reaction, they retreated. It was a battle for every small thing with them.

"Why don't you buy some white sarees for your mother?" said one knowledgeable old woman. "It's the custom and we have to change her saree." A white saree was the dress code for a widow. I had a problem even with the word widow being used for her.

"No, my father told her that she can wear coloured sarees," I bit back sharply. After much persuasion, Mother was convinced that Father would like to see her well-dressed as she always was. Consequently, she continued to wear the bright chiffon and georgette sarees that he had bought for her.

Lost and dazed, she had no energy to argue and she did as bade.

My brothers and I became incapable of any more emotional damage that blunted our senses for years to come. There was no time for grieving for there were unavoidable tasks waiting and unfinished businesses to be dealt with. I thought I had cried, mourned and grieved my share for a lifetime. I did not take any days off from the clinic after he passed away as I knew that the running of the clinic was most important to him. The clinic became an act of honour and loyalty to Father and that's how it remained for thirty-eight years.

I grew up overnight from a pampered 'doted upon daughter' to a woman of twenty-eight.

I wrote these lines a few days later:

Mustard Bloom

Mustard fields in celebration
Like a sea of bobbing heads
At a winter carnival
As we drove, we were
Together
The old times, years ago, you remembered
Fondly
The first car we had.
I looked out at the blinding
yellow shroud
Nailed to the vacant horizon
Like an extension of the sky
itself.
As I am alone today, you no more
I stand sobbing
Jaded, jaundiced tears
The yellow sleet flows
Like embalmed sunlight
I remember the mustard fields
Along with the pain of shared blooms
Dear Father!

My firstborn was just short of two months. I started driving to the clinic in my own car. Those were the longest, loneliest, emptiest drives of my life. This was the beginning of my fear of highway drives.

CHAPTER THREE

After the Accident

WHAT HAPPENED AFTER the accident was another tragedy that no one could anticipate. After the accident, my eldest brother moved into the posh farmhouse along with his wife and children in 1988. By this time, I was completely entrenched in the Kapashera way of life, working all days of the week. This was partly because most of my patients were factory workers, and Sunday was the only day they could come with their wives and families. If a worker took an hour off to visit my clinic, he would lose his daily wage or even be laid off. The other reason for attending Sunday clinic was that my husband would go to the hospital for his morning rounds to see his patients, so he wasn't home on Sundays anyway. Over the years, he rose to be a Professor and a faculty member and had to go for teaching rounds. The children got used to our Sunday routine, and it gave them space to do their own things and just be children. My heart yearned for the lazy lunches with pearls and wines. The ambience of the garden lunches was not for me now. Sundays made me the saddest as Delhi partied away. The sadness was for a life that I had foregone and the memory of Father that gnawed constantly.

The farm held many fond memories for me. I could almost feel Father's smile and his sure steps. I liked to walk the muddy pathways of the sprawling farm whenever I got a break from patients. The poplars and the silver oaks were taller and the underside of their leaves flickered like silverfish in the sunlight. Spring was worse on the sadness scale. As the first spring arrived just two months later, the poppies that Father had planted bloomed a bloody red and the candytuft looked a snowy white. The blooms may have looked pretty to some but for me they were heart-wrenching. The carnations that Father had bent over to tend to had grown taller and glistened in the sun with tearful eyes as they shed millions of coloured tears.

There were changes that caused tremors and sorrow in the idyllic life we had lived when Father was around. Wealth was a mundane, quiet presence that I had never even acknowledged. This was the first time that I grasped the enormity of the assets he had left and the influence it had on our lives.

Money is an excellent cleaver of people, I realised.

January 1986, soon after Father met his end on the road, was the year of the greatest apostasy for me. I saw strong bonds of relationships crumbling. Even as I experienced the grimness of poverty of my patients, I understood the havoc too much wealth could cause. The onslaught of excessive prosperity changed different people in different ways. Father left behind numerous factories, offices in every corner of the country, the farm and, of course, the family home. All this opulence ripped and exposed the frayed meshes of the family. I was saddened by this turn of events because I loved my brothers. Mother remained dazed and unresponsive for a long time for she knew of no world beyond her husband. She walked around looking miserable and trying to come to terms with the tragedy.

The room in the family home which Father had saved for me even after I got married found other uses by its new occupants. With every passing day I mourned Father even more, as I lost the home I had grown up in. However, Father's belief in me had given me so much strength that I could bear the destruction of a great family with silent grace.

My husband's father passed away just a year later, which was another tremor in our lives. The death of his father was distressful in itself but it was the events that followed which rendered us homeless, and more feuds and more angst clouded our existence.

Father had envisioned a bigger dream for me. He had constructed a mammoth building just yards away from my clinic.

"This will be your hospital," he had stated one day as he paced his farm. There was never a doubt or a hint of uncertainty in his statements. He was used to things being done his way. This building was only a hundred meters away from my small clinic.

My husband was similar to me in that he had no comity with money. This provided stability to our little family amongst the turmoil over the division of familial assets. We quietly made our new home in the big building that Father had built for us. That abandoned building did not ever house patients; it housed a family that was dear to him instead. Our son loved this house and christened it 'big house'. He could skate down the long, shiny passages shrieking with delight. He spent his summer vacations chasing his GI JOE planes in the long corridors and was happy to have many rooms to himself; which kid wouldn't? He had a shoe room, a toy room, a books room, a TV room and, of course, a bedroom. I am sure he carries pleasant memories of this huge building where he ran wild at three.

My husband and I accepted the fact that the big house was nothing like a conventional home. It had long stretches of endless rooms with a lighted corridor running between them. After all, it had been constructed to become a hospital. There was a huge hall as one entered, which was meant to be the reception and the general multipurpose area. We didn't have much in terms of worldly belongings, so the huge hall remained barren. There was no functional kitchen. We created our own kitchen by laying two tables in one of the rooms and a basic gas stove.

The days were fine but the building looked dark and gloomy in the evenings. Long corridors, rows of empty rooms, a large hall and an even larger basement all looked ominous after sunset. A small family of three sitting at their small dining table, trying to create cheerfulness in this huge building was poignant. Turning up the volume of the TV and lighting a few candles helped to create some sense of warm habitation. Two years later, in the 'big house', we were blessed with the prettiest baby girl ever. There was no doubt that dear Father was beaming at me and my family!

Home is where the heart is, I discovered, as we lived in this hospital building which was so unlike a regular home. In time, it became the sweetest and strangest home there could be.

There would be random snake sightings in the rooms, but my husband was fearless in dealing with these reptilian visits. The house grew on us, even as we climbed down on the social and economic ladder by a couple of notches, for who in the world lives in an abandoned hospital building? In spite of our coming down in life, we experienced a kind of quiet contentment which permeated our beings.

I knew that Father had really worked hard on constructing this for over two years. He had lofty dreams of opening a rural hospital in the summer of 1986. Had this hospital materialised, it would have been the best service to the rural folks for years to come. Even after thirty-eight years there is no hospital anywhere near. To my eternal regret, it was not to be. After the accident, neither my husband nor I were geared for such a tremendous responsibility, because running a hospital meant a lot of night calls, increased fear of litigation and even less time for the children. Moreover, my husband loved teaching so he had to be in a teaching hospital. The thought of letting down my father nagged me constantly for decades. After six years in this house we moved out into a proper home. The big hospital has lain quiet and uncomplaining for almost four decades now.

CHAPTER FOUR

Kalawati Saran Children's Hospital (KWSCH) 1982

THE MANDATORY ROTATING internships and the two six-month house jobs in Radiology and Paediatrics in 1981 exposed me to enough experience to deal with various illnesses to last me a lifetime. I realised that textbooks don't teach a fraction of the permutations that disease and the human body can conjure up. Working at KWSCH, I witnessed more cases than doctors from the developed world would come across in their whole career. I write that fact with great humility as India is a populous country and KWSCH was the largest children's tertiary care hospital in the country. Children who could not be treated in the remotest part of the country would find their way to the ER department of this hospital. I can never thank my luck enough that I chose paediatrics as my house job. Six months of experience here armed me with enough knowledge to pursue the GP practice I had been destined for. Sick children and babies who were preterm, bloated, limp, semi-conscious and almost dead, thronged its ER department, where they were examined, treated and then sent off to the various wards.

When the wards were filled with these sick children, one could see them overflowing in the corridors. There were times we had to put two or three children on one bed. Outside the wards, every inch of the hospital was occupied by mothers and other relatives who looked expectantly at anyone passing by, in a white coat. They sat with gloomy faces as they waited and hoped for miracles that would save their child. Everyone seemed to be waiting and praying.

Miracles were happening every moment; yet they were not enough. There were just too many sick children. Plaintive wails of the grieving parents would echo in different wards, down the corridors, and around the hospital as mothers moaned for the babies who could not make it. Death became such a frequent part of the day that it stopped bothering me after a while. It's wrong to say that because, no, it didn't stop bothering me. Every time I faced death, I would get that queasy feeling in the stomach. One learnt to live with the queasiness. This was the time my fellow interns and I learnt to be immune to sickness and tragedy. We tried not to let death affect our equanimity. This immunity from death was profound but did not make us invincible, as we wept silent tears and held the lump that formed in our throats, whenever a little baby was declared dead. A few of my colleagues even got to the stage where they could eat their lunch in the side rooms of the ward. I could never do that as the sickly smell of the wards overwhelmed me with nausea.

The large nursery (where the littlest ones were treated) was always full, and the newborns were discharged as soon as they could breathe without the ventilator. It was a collective effort of all doctors to remove as many babies from the ventilators as they could to make way for many more tiny lives that gasped for oxygen or IV lines. Some were born a tad early and weighed barely half a kilo, so they needed support until their lungs could gulp the air of the outside world on their own. The sweet, rancid smell of breast milk, wounds and sickness engulfed all the senses. It was nauseating initially, but then the stench became a normal smell in the memory. The best paediatricians in India hurried down the corridors as they rushed to a call for intubation or to resume an impossible IV line. The senior doctors I worked with in KWSCH were dedicated, hard-working and walking encyclopaedias of Paediatrics. In between their continuous forty-hour duties, they had to take undergraduate and postgraduate classes. To say that their academics were in top order would be an understatement.

Thinking back, I realise that it was a privilege to work there and to learn from the best.

It was disheartening to see that diseases that could be treated by a primary health worker in remote settings were neglected until they became life threatening. Why would a simple ailment like gastroenteritis cause a toddler to waver between life and death? A simple cough and cold led to pneumonia if treated indifferently and later could lead to meningitis. During the eighties, the infant mortality rate was high because most cases were brought in too late, when they were beyond treatment and hope. Such malaise and casual indifference in the 1980s, especially towards children, was appalling and unforgivable. There were just not enough doctors in the rural areas as every doctor aspired to be a super-duper specialist and work in the best hospitals, hence the grassroots levels did not have enough medical care. The same problem exists even today. Probably ninety percent of the sick people wouldn't need hospital admissions if they were provided decent medical care by a GP—a lowly GP like me.

Life was uncertain in those days and people believed that having more children created an insurance against being childless. I could have screamed in anger when some women, who already had three girls and one son, wanted another son. "What is one son?" they would say with a coy smile. "There should be at least two boys; one son is like having one eye." Sometimes I thought that the people who crowded our ERs, weeping and wailing, were devoid of any humane feelings. If one child died, there were plenty of other children at home or they quickly produced another one. This insecurity about life most likely explained why they were so productive in the reproduction field. That could be one of the reasons for India's galloping population.

The country seemed to be in shambles and each day in KWSCH made me realise that we lived in a third world country. Reading this memoir in a developed country, someone may wonder that if people had access to hospitals and specialist doctors, how was ours a third world country?

So here's the dichotomy. To give you an insight into many people's situations—if a dog bit a family of four, they would never be able to afford four anti-rabies shots because it would cost a full month's salary. Obviously, hard choices had to be made. The natural choice, of course, was for the son to receive the precious anti-rabies shot. The girls were left to the mercy of the divine. Poverty, sickness, malnourishment, illiteracy and the increasing millions of children, routed and negated any government plans. There were many generous and well-meaning plans for the underprivileged. Free vaccinations, free medical treatment, free birthing facilities, free schooling, free rations and free mid-day meals for all school children. The children received free textbooks and uniforms for school. Yet, these plans fell short. Very short!

As I mentioned earlier, the diseases we saw were different from the ones prevalent today. Cases of tetanus, rabies, pneumonia, dehydration, burns, head injuries and poisonings were common in the eighties. Wards were filled with complications of mumps and chickenpox.

The whoop of the diphtheria cough was exactly as the books described it and no one could mistake it for something else. With the advent of vaccines and the compliance of the patients, diphtheria, measles, and polio dwindled. Throughout the nineties, one could discern a downward trend in the cases of diphtheria and by the 2000s, the disease had vanished. These were the success stories of a third world country.

The hospital had a polio ward which held many children. They received the best care one could provide yet no one could blow a breath of life into those limp limbs that lay flaccid on the beds. Distressed parents searched our faces beseechingly for help, even though we looked helpless ourselves. In time we learnt to avoid their searching gaze and disheartened tears. There was no treatment. The disease occurred so insidiously. A child would go to bed with the legs kicking healthy but get up in the morning with flaccid limbs. I got many panic-stricken parents whose children had suddenly developed limp legs. It was polio that struck most insidiously. No amount of massaging or voodoo helped.

In 1995, India had over 50,000 cases of polio in a year. To call them cases would be insensitive as they were little kids and one could not walk away just referring to them as cases.

The relentless polio drive started in 1995 brought results almost two decades later. Funded by Rotary Clubs and WHO, this drive was the most successful in any country. I offered my clinic as a polio vaccine centre and two drops of the vaccine were given to hundreds of children for four decades in my clinic. My heart filled with joy when mothers with babies in arms came rushing for the drops. I kept sweets for the children and used this opportunity to check other vaccinations too. With regular awareness and polio vaccination drives, cases of polio reduced drastically and India became polio free in the year 2011. It was a big victory as over 70 percent cases of polio in the world were from this sub-continent.

I am one of the few doctors in 2020 who saw rabies cases in her lifetime. For those who aren't aware, rabies is debilitating or fatal, yet there were no stringent rules in place for neutering strays. Rabies-ridden stray dogs teemed the streets, unfettered, which caused the disease to spread. These strays established their presence by barking in unison in every locality, and they bit anyone in any place at any time without cause or reason. The incidence was more in children as children were more likely to wake sleeping dogs in the street and play with them with blissful naivety. People were nonchalant and apathetic towards this grave disease that came unannounced as they thought that it happened only to others and that it was a God-given curse. Vaccination was not acceptable due to its high cost and the inconvenience of getting five doses. Probably, the cost was the biggest deterrent, and the fact that the earlier subcutaneous version was administered in the abdomen was intimidating for most. As a result, the rabies wards were never empty.

As junior residents, we admitted a substantial number of tetanus cases too. It feels strange to not have seen or heard of a tetanus case in so many years. It was a nightmare to admit those children because they were brought in taut, and contorted in spasms. In the eighties, a tetanus shot was not a normal medication which was a pity. A small injury caused by an innocent-looking nail, knife or a rusty nut, or even an innocuous fall on the road could cause such a fatal blow. The tetanus jab cost just ten rupees and was affordable for most families, but they would not take the injection. In my clinic, many years later, no matter how hard I tried to convince my patients, people never agreed to getting a tetanus shot for the confidence of the healthy is difficult to deal with.

"It's just a small cut," some would say. Awareness and compliance was low. Finally, with awareness and better education in the 2000s, it is heartening to see people coming on their own and asking for a tetanus shot even for small needle injuries. How it happened, I cannot tell, but tetanus faded out happily.

One can breathe easy because a lot of good changes have occurred in medicine in the last three decades. The fact that the burns wards have just a few beds these days speaks well of the progress we have made to lower the child mortality rate from preventable diseases. The wood fires which were common in homes and were set up at floor level saw many scalds and burns because the mother cooked with her toddler in her lap. Babies were brought in with scalds and burns caused by boiling water, spilled tea or cinder burns. I would be totally distraught on

Diwali night as kid after kid got admitted with burns caused by firecrackers. With the new piped gas and compressed gas in every home, cooking on table tops became the norm and new rules banning firecrackers reduced the incidence of burns.

Timely treatment of influenza prevented pneumonia and meningitis. With increased urbanisation, snake, monkey, rodent and insect bites became rare.

In February 1982, not long after I started working at KWSCH, I met my husband-to-be. He was pursuing MS surgery at the time and was posted in the Paediatric surgery unit. Our first dinner date is quite a story. We were both on night duty and had decided on walking down to a nice Chinese restaurant in Connaught place. My colleague agreed to cover up for me while I was away. All was set and I waited for him to come to the paediatrics ward. Minutes ticked by and I kept waiting. Persistent peeping down the long corridor didn't help either. I decided to go to his Operation Theatre which was some distance away. On reaching his OT, I saw him sitting in his scrubs eyeing a vague, sticky mass on a tray in front of him.

He looked up and seeing me looking at him said, "Look what I operated on today!" I tried to match his enthusiasm but the mass on the table looked disgusting. I feigned interest and asked, "What's that?"

"It's a ball of worms," he informed eagerly. "This kid of seven came in with acute pain in his abdomen. I diagnosed and operated."

To my horror, he pulled the worms apart from the mass, one by one, with his gloves on, of course. Like noodles they hung limp as he counted them one by one. He was clearly in no hurry and was enjoying the spoils of his surgery even as my stomach churned. I knew dinner was definitely not on the plate now, especially noodles. He had obviously forgotten the dinner date in the exuberance of a new surgeon. "I need to get back," I said hurriedly and scampered down to my ward ready to throw up.

After a short engagement period came the phase of being newly-married. For doctors there are no personal phases or milestones. The patients, the wards, the duties continued. Back-to-back, thirty-six hour duties with fifteen hours off in between, which was the norm for all doctors was my routine. My husband left for England soon after we were married. He hoped to pursue the surgery fellowship, the mandatory FRCS, which every self-respecting surgeon coveted. I was at a loose end. Once he left, it was obvious that I was left with plenty of free evenings. I volunteered to do the night duties of other interns and offered to work on all public holidays, festivals and weekends to keep myself from moping around and missing him. This made me immensely popular with the other interns as they could stay at home on all holidays and festivals while this arrangement provided me with a safe haven to retreat to. I remember when it was my first Diwali as a married girl, I was miffed about something in my new home and I jumped at the chance of doing my friend's night duty in the ward just to get away; she was happy as working on a Diwali night was the worst duty for any doctor. As I mentioned, I was miffed and it was natural that I did not tell anyone at home about my Diwali night duty. So no one knew where I was on that night; I just went missing. What a furore it caused in both my 'new' marital home and my own home! Well, I was young and can smile about it today.

Each day, the OPD (Outpatient Department) had more than fifty admissions during the day and fifty at night, but the ones admitted at night were usually the really sick ones.

The heroism in Kalawati was a daily affair. The joy of witnessing a child with an absent pulse, suddenly letting out a long wail after vigorous CPR (Cardiopulmonary resuscitation) is incomparable to any joy I have experienced. All these procedures and the handling of little children gave me a taste for real medicine. As trainees, we were guided by senior resident doctors, and the babies who had suspected meningitis were given a lumbar puncture (LP) test, which involved putting a needle in the lumbar spine and withdrawing the cerebrospinal fluid. It seemed impossible at first, but after observing the senior residents and how easily they managed to do it, I ventured to perform this procedure. The first one I did was a nightmare because I thought the baby might die with my long needle, but later I ended up doing five to six a day. It was disappointing when the fluid wouldn't fill up the needle, but the senior residents were kind and forgiving and encouraged us to try again.

Many children came in with gastroenteritis, but it was not just any gastroenteritis. It was the gastroenteritis that killed thousands of children every single day. They were severely dehydrated, hadn't passed urine for a day, their fontanelles were sunken and the skin hung loosely around their tiny bodies. The babies were so weak that they looked like newborn pigeons with shrivelled faces, scrawny necks and deep, sunken eyes. As most of them had collapsed veins, starting an intravenous drip was an impossible task, yet we continued to try until we found a good vein, even if it was in their scalp. Just a hundred millilitres of fluid could be life-saving, so we tried relentlessly to find veins.

Holding and treating these sick children in KWSCH made me comfortable with their smallness and frailness and helped me save thousands of children from dying in my clinic. I overcame the usual fear most doctors have when they see newborns or sick children.

One evening in August of 1983, the emergency had been exceptionally busy in the hospital and I was on night duty with the senior resident. A weeping woman rushed into the ER and unwrapped a baby from her endless folds and put it on the table. The senior resident looked at the baby and then looked at me and shook his head to signal that the baby was dead.

"Amma, the baby is no more; take it home." He looked at the mother as if in apology.

"Please help, please help, doctor." I could see that the senior resident was wavering.

"Let me try intracardiac adrenaline," he said with a resolve. When one knows that the battle is lost, there comes a new strength and a new fearlessness because one knows that there is nothing more to be lost. He quickly told the nurse to get an adrenaline injection. As he injected the adrenaline into the dead baby's heart, I kept doing CPR. We continued fighting the battle because we had to and not because we expected to win. After a few moments, the baby's eyes flickered and it let out a loud cry. We looked at each other in jubilation. That evening in KWSCH helped me to save a life ten years later in my remote, rural clinic.

The ward visits were a delight every morning, especially when the children and their mothers welcomed me with bright smiles. They waited for me to walk into the ward and the mothers would fold their hands and bend down to touch my feet in gratitude. Strangers touching my feet made me uncomfortable, yet it reinforced the feeling that I was finally a respected doctor.

CHAPTER FIVE

All about Radiology

THE FIRST SIX months of my residency were in Radiology. My reasonable score allowed me to choose any subject for residency, but I was so sure about pursuing Paediatric practice that no other subject interested me. Yet, I needed a six-month filler, so it was Radiology for me. Besides, I got engaged in February of 1982 and working in Radiology seemed to be a no-brainer since there would be no night duties, no emergencies and it was a laid-back department. I could indulge in all the dating time I wished for. What else could one want? All my friends wondered about the sanity of my choice. Who in the world does a Radiology house job out of free will when there are more exciting choices available? I never gave it much thought and just flowed into it whimsically. It was like one of those electives that are unsubstantial but people take just for accumulating credits. I was sure of the fun time to be had as there was obviously no useful learning involved here. How wrong I was!

As it turned out, this serendipitous choice of Radiology proved to be a godsend for the career I was destined to pursue. I remember we had a Moral Science book in school that was treated as a Bible in my Irish convent. It had stories from the Bible and the one that made an indelible dent in my receptive fifteen-year-old brain were the lines:

God Writes Straight With Crooked Lines.

These were just lines that we had to learn for tests and never seemed too profound at that time. Years later, when I was all alone in my small clinic, I had my own X-ray machine and a row of patients who waited for their X-ray reports. I sat bemused and remembered those lines in Moral Science. If the clinic had not happened, Radiology would have had no relevance in my life. How did I stumble onto it is a question that baffles me even forty years later? A quiet department, with very few staff, it was strategically placed at the end of the hospital. It had no glamour attached to it while Surgery, Medicine, Gynaecology and Paediatrics were residencies that were coveted and respected. It was strange how with all my uppityness, I walked straight into Radiology.

Initially, it was a reprieve not to be running around like an intern. As everyone knows, interns are the fittest people on earth because it is they who are summoned to deliver blood samples or to get reports that need to be procured from the path lab a couple of miles away. They run to deliver slides to the histology lab, to arrange blood transfusions, to retrieve old records from the archives, to summon the relatives waiting outside for news of their patient and whatever jobs the peons would refuse to do. All odd jobs were relegated to the interns. At times I wished to be in the peon's shoes as he could refuse to do certain things and was way more respected than an intern. I remember I would wear my running shoes to work as each department was miles away from the other. “The slides are lying on the side table,” a stern voice would ring down the ward, “can you please run and hand them in the histology lab?”

“Of course I will.” I would begin my sprint. After all, I had my running shoes on. There would be many such sprints on any single day. It kept us fit and slim. Who had the time for gyms and workouts with back to back twelve-hour shift duties?

In Radiology, it felt good to be a resident doctor, even a junior one, as one could dress up nicely and there was no need for those undignified sprints. Hence, I could blow dry my hair and wear the beautiful blouses that hung in my wardrobe and walk delicately in my high-heeled shoes. I loved having a designated chair and a desk of my own in the department.

Father was proud of my achievements and walked with a perpetual smile on his face. He waited every morning for me at the breakfast table as I flung my white coat over the chair and joined him.

“How is the hospital?” He would smile affectionately at me, curious to know about the wards and the patients. After breakfast he watched me drive off in my brand new Fiat.

Sadly, our dates were not as frequent as I expected as my fiancé was too busy learning the intricacies of surgery. Obviously, I was never in a hurry to go anywhere and after a while, everyone realised my willingness to do any extra work thrown my way. I was a willing junior resident so the senior residents rewarded me with endless samosas and tea. My conscientiousness gave them opportunities to ramble around in Connaught Place markets, eating, shopping and ogling at the modern non-medico girls from the university campus. They checked on me a few times for any blunders, but once they were sure that my reports were correct, they left it all to me.

I loved the respectful way the paramedical staff wished me good morning every day. That was a far cry from being an intern where we had to cajole and hammer the paramedics for any work to be done. The paramedical staff wondered about me as I caught their furtive glances and inquisitive looks. They speculated about the quiet worker, newly-engaged, who would not leave with the rest of the staff at the stroke of four. They displayed their admiration and joy by offering me endless cups of coffee and cookies.

Gazing at the mysterious dark X-rays that held signs of disease, I savoured my time in the department as I sat for hours in front of the lighted X-ray boxes and reported the mysterious films taken during the day. The X-rays that had been requested from the various departments of the hospital would come to the Radiology Department to be reported. The diagnosis of the disease was dependent on my reports which were eagerly awaited by all doctors and patients. It was a heady thought to be able to give a verdict! What, little me doing all this? I worked tirelessly as if driven by an unknown urgency. I learnt about Barium studies for ailments of the gut and IVPs (Intravenous Pyelograms) for renal stones. All these procedures seemed fascinating to me. The sudden affinity for X-rays, cannulas and ultrasound-guided injection of the dye was a surprise. Why I developed a love for X-rays was a wonder.

However, the best thing I learnt there were the Hysterosalpingograms (HSGs), which were done predominantly for infertility cases. I enjoyed watching the dye fill the uterus and the fallopian tubes as it showed up in the X-rays. It just made invisible things visible. Sometimes I performed four to five HSGs a day in that quiet department. When I look back on those years, it's inevitable to believe that I was just a pawn in a larger game. The larger game was the clinic that was to be. The Paediatrics and Radiology residency both trained me for the more significant role I was destined to play for the rest of my life. Even though Kapashera and the rural practice were never on my horizon during my time at medical school, yet I learnt those very skills which held me well for decades and became the strong point of my profession as a GP.

To completely denounce an unfamiliar subject is silly, I learnt. I always tell my children that learning is never too small or in vain. However insignificant it may seem, it has to be cherished.

The clinic became a reality in 1983. Besides the usual children and women ailments, it was the chronic coughs and breathlessness cases that bothered me. There was no laboratory doing chest X-rays anywhere near the clinic. Father understood my frustration in not being able to fully care for these patients and as only a father can, he talked me into getting my own X-ray machine. I gave in, knowing that I would have to give in anyway. In a matter of days, I had this 60 MA beauty sitting in a small outhouse at the farm. Promptly, he built another room to house the new Siemens machine and, of course, a big board came up proclaiming loud and clear 'Dr Jindal's X-Ray clinic'. I smile to think that Father received vicarious pleasure in putting up these large boards. I understand his enthusiasm even as I glow proudly at my children's smallest achievements. Every time I walk into the clinic, I look at these big boards and chuckle to myself and I know Father is proud of me. The X-ray envelopes got printed and I had a functional X-ray set up. For someone who did not want to do Radiology, I knew I was being tried over and over again in resilience. Destiny was having a field day at my cost. This was the year 1985. If I had to single out one thing that changed lives in Kapashera and in the villages around, it would be the X-ray machine. The inflow of patients with chronic cough and fever increased as word about the machine got around.

In the early years it was only used for the injury cases to diagnose fractures due to the large number of industrial accidents. I diagnosed fractures, suspected and real. Since there was a lot of industrial activity in this region, with little care for safety and no fear of litigation, it was obvious that industrial accidents were a common occurrence. Road accidents were my love and hate interest. Since my clinic was at a crossing, there were many accidents, big and small. Victims would just walk in with bleeding cuts and bruises and lots of moaning. To vindicate Father dying on the road, I treated all road accidents for free. To clean up their wounds slowly and lovingly gave me a kind of comfort because I hadn't been able to help Father as he lay on the road, bleeding and dying. For me it was a labour of love and felt that I was tending to my father's wounds.

The accidents were brought in with much fanfare with the patient bleeding and surrounded by a conglomeration of the co-workers or passers-by. "Please have a look, doctor, he is badly hurt," they would expect instant attention. "So much blood, doctor." At times a cop would accompany the injured man and the sheepish-looking rash driver. The unsaid word of law was that the culprit would pay the entire medical bill for the injury and shell out a few extra hundred rupees to the victim. Once outside the clinic, the cop would receive another hundred for his services and for not making it into a medico-legal case. The arrangement was good for all.

I could manage most of the injuries in my clinic. Some injured patients needed an X-ray, which was an instant service in my clinic. With the Radiology training, it was easy to diagnose the wet films within minutes. Very few of them had to be referred to a tertiary care hospital.

The thought bothered me constantly, that if most illnesses could be managed by a GP in a small clinic, why were the big hospitals bulging with patients and why did they rush to specialists for minor ailments? If only small GP clinics received more respect, many more doctors would venture into this tremendous service.

The Tuberculosis spate drowned me in the eighties and well into the 2000s. The path to diagnosing and treating had been paved by the Radiology residency. Whenever a patient came with a history of loss of weight and mild fever, I would advise an X-ray.

What is the magic line they say these days? '*Follow your heart*'. Let me tell you one thing about this most overrated advice of the century. Following your heart is a complete eyewash.

I wasted decades disgruntled, dissatisfied and discontented and wallowing in the thought that I could not follow my heart; it was the feeling that overpowered me most at that time. Years later, when wisdom dawned, I knew that I had got the best career anyone could hope for; a gratifying platform that was so humbling. I also knew that I was the privileged one, not the pitiable one.

CHAPTER SIX

Learning and Unlearning 1983-2020

AFTER THE HIGHLY academic and specialised environment of KSCH, I stepped foot in Kapashera. The first ten years were my primitive phase as I reeled under a cultural, personal and professional shock. I was fresh off the boat with a new degree, zero experience, a new unfamiliar terrain and a brand-new marriage. All these changes were unimaginable for a twenty-five-year-old medical graduate. I had to stop thinking about the life that could have been had we managed to get to England.

A private practice is like the first dive into the deep sea. GPs are vulnerable as they are completely alone in their clinic with no one to turn to for help or advice. The sole GP doesn't have the backing of paramedical and other medical staff and no luxury of a second opinion. All good deeds and saved lives are forgotten in a moment if one patient, just one patient succumbs to his sickness. A nemesis for any doctor. Most GP clinics function with basic facilities but my clinic had to be run on an extremely low budget too. The only redeeming factor was that I could always call my husband whenever I felt the need for free medical advice. It is natural for GPs to make up for the lack of equipment by developing their own faculties and the sixth senses to diagnose disease. Learning the ropes of a full-blown clinical practice was like walking a tightrope because for me the clinic was a completely alien world. It was too rural and my patients were too illiterate.

Kapashera and all its satellite villages were infested with toothy, unkempt quacks dressed in faded loose kurtas. And I was a young woman wearing nice fashionable tops, my hair styled perfectly. A totally unexpected and unwelcome presence, or so I thought. There was a degree of wariness in people as they peeped into the clinic and walked out. In spite of the ones that left, there was not a single day that the four benches outside were not full. My waiting room never did any waiting ever, because for every one patient walking out there were five who entered, yet I felt humiliated in a strange way for it seemed like rejection. After the peeping and leaving kept repeating itself many times over the next few weeks, the thought kept me awake at nights trying to figure out why people did not enter the clinic. I assumed that it could have been because I was a lone female in a male-dominated, rural milieu. Constant feedback from my regular patients reinforced the belief that it was mostly due to my age—people assumed that I had no experience as a doctor.

The real reason revealed itself when an obliging patient said, "It is because of these clothes as you don't look like a doctor."

"What's wrong with my clothes?"

He drew my attention gently to my shirt and pants, "You

look too modern and people don't connect with you, they think you are an outsider." I was mortified! The other patients were right about my age and experience; now maybe my clothes too were a problem. The point hit right home.

That moment I knew I had to make myself look older and more experienced, and more rural. Easy! Discarding the pants and pretty tops, I scoured the markets with my new sister-in-law and bought a couple of six-yard cotton sarees. She also advised me to tie up my hair and taught me to bun it tightly. I inspected the quick transformation in the mirror and smiled with satisfaction as I looked ten years older. I acquired a new confidence and authority overnight and strode into my clinic with the aplomb of a senior doctor. Soon I was congratulating myself when not one patient peeped in and left.

Gradually, the saree became my clinic garb. If ever a gaze wandered away from my face to elsewhere, my sarees became thicker, the blouses became longer and the necklines became higher. I wanted to be taken seriously and had to prove that I was not some callow doctor straight out of medical school. I was not here to look glamorous and no matter how thick and coarse, a saree imparts an unmatched elegance and authority.

I need to stress upon the way men dress. Has anyone ever seen a man with the top button open, his hair falling over his face or his biceps showing, at his work place? If we want a fair playing field at work places, let's play fair. I see many women wearing low necks, tight tops with seductive hair strands falling all around. Why should anyone wear such clothes to work? I know I will be trolled forever for stating these facts. The workplace and social settings are different. If women take away the attention from their own anatomy, no one else will pay any attention to it too. I covered myself with thick cotton sarees so as not to draw attention to my body.

As years went by, I revived my dormant fashion sense and hunted the best shops for unusual sarees and bought the rich Indian hand-woven ones from different states of India. The weaves of every state are different and I lapped them up. In the summers, the silks were replaced by the cotton ones that kept me cool in the Indian heat. The cotton ones needed to be starched daily. Ironing a crisp, starched cotton saree is an art form in itself, but I was lucky to have an ironing man who enjoyed ironing my sarees each day on his table outside my home. These ironing men and women or 'presswalas', as they are called, are present in every colony. They iron shirts, blouses and trousers for just a small amount and no one really needs a dry cleaner.

"Let's play the game perfectly," I said to myself every morning, as I draped my sarees with perfect, blade-sharp pleats. I would pull out a saree, drape it, make my prim bun and put a decorative bindi onto my forehead. It was a drill that was adeptly executed. There was no preening or gazing into the mirror, for vanity was irrelevant in Kapashera. I learnt that the villagers spoke about this quiet doctor in Kapashera, who always looked elegant in her sarees and a bun. Bits and pieces of the grapevine found their way to my ears, that women travelled long distances just to have a look at my crisp, cotton sarees.

In spite of the success of my sarees, deep down in my heart, I longed for the suave pencil skirts and heels I would have worn in London, with my heels clicking as I went about hospital work. Loss of pencil skirts was a big regret that haunted me for years. I knew I was meant to be in London. I daydreamed about the red buses of London and the rush of the big, beautiful city. I longed to style my hair into the blunt bob that I loved and craved the fairy lights at romantic garden parties.

In the times of COVID-19, my husband accompanied me to the clinic on Sundays. He sat quietly and read his book as I filed through my patients. I knew he came just to check if I was keeping my promise of not physically examining the patients and wearing my full protective gear—a mask, a face shield, two layers of gowns and, of course, gloves. Given my habit of listening to my patients for hours, he helped me put the benches outside the clinic on the sidewalk to avoid infection and write down the treatment without any physical examination. This can happen only in Kapashera as nowhere else in the world would patients sit on the sidewalk. It's almost like telemedicine, but my patients find it reassuring to see me in person and believe that I can diagnose their illness just by looking at them, which is true to a certain extent because after decades I am better at diagnosing 'just like that'.

One day, my husband sat in the clinic and checked his phone for zero messages for he is a nonbeliever of the benefits of social groups. All the years that I have known him, he has been impregnable, stoical and impassive to a fault. No one could ever mistake his silence for a 'nothing to say' silence. His erudite silence commands people to tiptoe around him and speak in hushed whispers. I am sure that it is not something that he has adopted just to scare people away; it's just the way he is. Maybe his manner seeped into my subconscious behaviour and I got used to scurrying back into my comfort zone at the slightest hint of disagreement. I don't think he was aware of me pre-empting his displeasure. As he sat there lost in his phone, one of my regular patients sneaked over to him and said, "Doctor, I have a fever."

I didn't know whether to be annoyed or amused. It was obvious that the patient had assumed that he could get better advice from a male doctor.

My husband looked up from his phone and frowned with confusion because fevers were not his territory since he was a surgeon.

"I have aches here also," continued the man rubbing his tummy, "and here," pointing at his head.

"She is the doctor here, not me," said my husband, pointing towards me and dismissing the man without a second thought. I knew it was not a compliment to me; it was just that he didn't want to be bothered by a fever patient. In most parts of the world, men were doctors and women were nurses. Period! To come across a doctor who was a female rocked their conditioned gender biases. There can never be a female surgeon. If there is, it has to be specified to the patients and to their relatives before the surgery. There have been cases where patients have arisen from the operating table and left as soon as they realised that a female would be performing the operation.

Most of my friends and colleagues moved away from me due to my lack of specialisation and running an insubstantial rural clinic. I stopped keeping track of them as some had moved abroad and were engrossed in practising high-end medicine. My dreams of going to the UK and of becoming the best paediatrician ever had quietly funnelled their way into the dark reality of the clinic. At times, it felt that I had been sucked into this dismal whirlpool totally unprepared, and I had accepted that there was no turning back.

Complete erasure of our past life ought to be an option. I wished to turn back and take the road not taken and start over again, just like everyone else; but everyone knows that there is no turning back or hoping for a second chance.

It was my belief that I was doing good to my patients that kept me going. After all, people visited my clinic from faraway places and even from other states. Some of them came straight from the train station with their bags. Some who required longer treatment rented rooms in nearby Samalkha and stayed until I declared them fit to return.

I received idolisation, affection and monetary benefits from my patients as I continued my pursuit of excellence with whatever resources and ability I had. The devotion my patients had for me was terrifying in its enormity. I wished that I could be like the other doctors who just see patients perfunctorily and send them home with a prescription. I was being weighed down by the reverential bowing and the touching of my feet. I longed for indifference in my patients because indifference or simple acceptance is sometimes better than reverence. I knew that the higher the pedestal one is raised to, the greater would be the fall. This fear kept me on tenterhooks all those years in Kapashera. Glorification brings the hazard of condemnation by even mildly disgruntled patients. Good communication and connectedness with the patients was a self-preservation tactic and a reasonable defense to avoid any humiliation.

Every day was a challenge because every human body is different and each patient responds differently to the same regimen of treatment. Every patient presents different permutations and combinations of signs and symptoms. Consequently, it was natural that I was learning with every patient. The number of different diseases in my oeuvre kept me on my toes for decades. My husband's sagacity kept me from losing mine in the face of the unnatural veneration that came my way.

There were times when I had a high fever and could barely walk, yet I sat at my table examining patients, trying to look as invincible as possible. Like most humans, I too had my share of flu, backaches, headaches, pregnancies, tummy upsets and everything else, but unlike most humans, I never allowed myself a day off.

Even though I lacked paediatric specialisation, gynaecology expertise, surgical prowess and fancy machines for diagnosis, I had no need for them because the number of people who waited eagerly for my attention was overwhelming. All I had to do was to talk and listen to my patients, and be compassionate and honest and involved with them. I just needed to be there! It certainly was not asking too much from me. It was a decent enough arrangement. There was no sceptre of a boss to measure my performance or take stock of my effectiveness. I was my own yardstick which was worse as self-flagellation was my favourite pastime.

When I listened to my patients, it felt as if the world stood still and the patient before me became the most important person in the world. The patient could have been an emaciated rickshaw-puller or a portly landowner in his brand new SUV flashing his wads of cash. It didn't matter who they were or where they came from; they were all important to me. I was always interested in their stories about infidelity, physical abuse, marital rape, and the abuse of young girls by the people they trusted the most. My mind became a storehouse for these endless tales.

For me, talking to a patient was never just a medical

consultation, it was a project. My involvement in those tales was a catalyst between me and my practice. In hindsight, I learnt a lot about the diagnosis of many mysterious illnesses from these narratives. I also learnt that if one can cure the mind, the body heals on its own. At times, I knew there was a long queue of patients in the outside waiting room, yet, I did not hurry through the patient who sat in front of me. They waited patiently as they were sure that they would get their fair share of time too.

I observed the patients without a hint of embarrassment and stored every expression and twitch of the face in the 'save mode'. Of course, I told myself that the reason for my unabashed observation was to diagnose and I wanted to bring about a change in their lives, but how was that possible if I wasn't at one with them?

There were many non-medical reasons for my observation too. Nowhere does the Hippocratic Oath define the length of time one can observe a patient. I observed their faces maybe a tad more than I needed to as a physician, and I hoarded the faces and the stories. I may be held guilty of being more interested in my patients' lives than was necessary on medical grounds. I simply loved the patients and their exotic stories, and knew they would later figure in my paintings. Art was also something I accidentally fell into for I had not planned on becoming an artist. From very humble beginnings as an artist, I moved forward in the most unintentional and undesigned manner. I suffered from a dichotomy of loyalty between being a medico and an artist. I beheld my patients in all their beauty, their ugliness, their calluses, and their warts as I tried to decipher the symptoms and find a cure for them.

In 1995, I had my first art show as a professional painter.

The faces I painted made everyone curious. They wanted to know why I painted only faces. What was my muse? Some people tell me to move on from painting faces, but where do they want me to move to? I do not know any other world besides these faces. I have lived my life with these faces and I have looked at them until their essence soaked into my being. There were times when my clinic became an artist's studio and I absorbed every curve of the cheek, every ridge of the nose, and pried through their facades to get to their thoughts.

My interest in other people's lives and their adulation in return was the symbiotic arrangement that sustained me for three and a half decades as I flailed amidst regrets, doubts and dismay. At what point the clinic became a sustaining need for me, I don't know. Whenever I glanced at the people on the wooden benches who waited patiently for hours for their turns, I knew I was doing good and changing the world even if in a small way. I felt needed and special. Their tales helped me to overcome the silent vacuum that my existence had become bereft of lunches, parties and all social interactions.

Going out of my way to help them even if it meant counselling them for education, financial matters, marital problems or advice on drug addiction became imperative. The redness or blueness on the face, neck and abdomen indicated physical abuse and the gaping wounds on their delicate parts disturbed me every time I saw them. Nonetheless, the cause of their wounds had to be deduced in silence because none of the women ever admitted that they had been beaten. After all, their husband was their God, so how could they incriminate him? As a result, I learnt to provide the treatment in silence without any mention of the cause. I simply wrote whatever medical history the patient gave me and pretended to believe it, even though both of us knew the true reason for their injuries. If I quizzed them a bit longer, their eyes would well up with agonised tears, so after some time, I learnt to accept their silence. However, sometimes they did ask for advice about how they could avoid the physical abuse. I tried to reason with their husbands, albeit without much success. At times persuading, fear of the police and fear of society helped in a few cases. Even if just one woman was spared from being abused, I could sleep in peace.

Some of the men who visited me as patients or with spouses had come to my clinic decades earlier as little boys in their mother's arms. They looked up to me and they remembered that they had circled my table for the little sweets kept in my drawer. It was unbelievable that those cute little boys had turned into wife batterers. Counselling them was easier as they were more amenable to my advice. At times, they would stand outside the clinic and not come in as they were unable to look me in the eye. When I called them in they would abashedly agree to stop the horrific behaviour.

As the eighties turned into the nineties and the new millenium dawned, my patients too changed with the times. India transformed from a stagnant to a developing economy and was on its way to becoming a global country. A new affluence saw more patients walking in. The expanding villages contributed a large number of patients. They were more than I could handle with the present set-up. I needed more staff to deal with the increasing numbers. Sundari and Sonam were recruited from nearby Samalkha to aid the earlier two, Roopa and Roopali. It was a sheer coincidence that all four names meant pretty. The irony was that the girls were getting good grades yet were made to drop out of school to supplement the family income. Their brothers continued schooling even though they barely made the pass grade. The boys were born blessed and ready to lap up the privileges of being a male.

Kapashera remained a rural, forgotten place for the rest of the world for years till the land boom happened. It was as if the sun was reluctant to rise here because every sunny day brought in dehydrated kids who could barely survive. The rain didn't know how to cast its monsoon magic here because all it did was make uncouth, ungraceful puddles. The reckless sheets of rain led to leaking roofs and overflowing drains. Families crouched under lonesome beams to stay dry. I was used to happy seasons in my life. The same seasons arrived in Kapashera with a different meaning. Its surrounding hamlets too were entrenched in squalidity and vacuity. I saw and understood the look of dread that clouded the faces of these villagers as the clouds filled the skies. The monsoon rains that had me singing and dancing my heart out would cause sleepless nights for most people in Kapashera. The primitive drains would overflow and the sewage would enter homes. The villagers spent entire days throwing bucketfuls of the blackish slush out from their bedrooms. I knew these details as my staff girls took a day off to do this task. They had a constant strained look on their young faces. "All the drain water has ruined our clothes and our bedding," rued Roopa. I could imagine a small home full of drain water, dark and damp, with no electricity. A small candle probably sufficed to see the level of the water and any creeping rodents.

"All our curtains and woollens are also wet," Sonam would pitch in ruefully.

"Ok, you can go a bit early," was all I could offer in terms of sympathy.

With so much acceptance amidst squalor, I knew I had no business moaning about the lack of beauty and ambience in my life. Father's beautiful farm was an oasis in the grimy and wretched environs that surrounded the clinic. The initial horror and disgust gradually changed to acceptance of a sad reality as I set about to make it better. I knew I could make lives better by advising them about better drainage and plumbing.

I added another room for procedures. I knew I had to move with the times. The doorway to my clinic was comparatively small. Once one entered, it fanned out to large open rooms. I kept it small even when I extended the clinic years later. There was a reason for the humble entry. Father had converted the guard room outside the farm into my clinic. Guard rooms have small doorways to restrict entry. It was a narrow wooden door. "It's teak wood," Father had said proudly the day it was installed.

The silver lining was that this door faced the east where the first morning rays entered the clinic lightning it up in more ways than one. I remember the first day when I had sat in front of the holy fire grumpily while the sunlight had poured in right through the small doorway. It fell on the benches, it fell on the people sitting on the benches and it lit up the room in a warm light. Ever since, I had become superstitious about this doorway. My waiting room has always been full of patients all these thirty-eight years. A few years back when I renovated my clinic, although the clinic faced the road and I had a choice of installing the latest, sliding glass doors, I chose not to change anything about this small doorway as an ode to Father.

From a newly-married couple, we grew into a middle-aged duo and our family grew from two sweet little infants to two young, independent adults. My son flew to the USA for his undergraduate degree. My husband and I dropped him off at the beautiful campus of UVA (University of Virginia). It was exciting to do up his dorm room, buying bed sheets, a book rack, a bath caddy, a comforter and a table fan from *Bed, Bath and Beyond*. I realised the depth of Father's joy at my clinic when my own children grew up and I experienced the same intense elation when my son was selected as the best student in senior school. I could not contain my tears when we walked the special carpet laid out for the parents of meritorious kids. I felt the same overwhelming joy that I had seen in Father's eyes that first day of the clinic in 1983. As my son walked towards his classroom, my heart was overwhelmed with joy seeing the spring in my son's step and the dreams that filled his eyes.

Five years later, my little baby girl too flew off to the USA. For a second time, we travelled to drop her off and we made the mandatory trip to *Bed, Bath and Beyond*. When we came back to an empty nest, my husband became busy in his surgical career, becoming the best surgeon there could be, and I, well I continued with my clinic.

CHAPTER SEVEN

Quacksalvers and Voodoo

THE FRUSTRATION I felt due to my own lack of resources was abated by the knowledge that medical facilities were non-existent in the area. Whatever little I was providing exceeded the best they were getting. I knew that armed with just one stethoscope and my training, I was far better than the best quack around the whole area.

The place was infested with quacks. They were local guys and people had faith in them. They looked like the locals and spoke their language. I faced tough competition from them for many years. I was the outsider, so it was I who had to prove myself. The quacks had always been there and were trusted. It's incredible that these quacks abound even in this age of modernity and have a robust following. Their small, dingy clinics have serpentine queues even today.

I heard stories about how they gave injections through the sleeves. Once, I asked a patient to roll up his sleeve for a tetanus shot. He looked queerly at me and said, "Dr Biswas gives it through the sleeve, you too give it the same way." I learnt that a single needle was used for all patients. It was discarded only by the end of the day, maybe not. It was an uphill task to explain to each patient the risk that the quack was subjecting them to. Obviously, the quack wasn't aware about the hazards of acquiring hepatitis A and AIDS from the use of the same needle and many other diseases. After all, he was illiterate and blissful in his ignorance.

Stories of this 'doctor' who would take X-rays for three rupees each bothered me. The cost of the X-ray film itself was fifty rupees in the eighties. I wondered how anyone could manage an X-ray for three rupees. "One hundred rupees for one X-ray!" exclaimed a patient.

"That is the minimum I can charge," I reasoned earnestly.

"How come Dr Shambhu does it in three rupees?"

I had to use my staff's wisdom and sleuthing abilities to get to the bottom of this so sent Meera for a recce of the quack's clinic. This was my only recourse to learn the ways of the village. The resourceful 'doctor' had an old fridge which served as an X-ray machine. He would make the patient stand in front of it and close the door with a snap. X-ray done! He would buy old films from hospitals and hand them to the patients.

An old fridge was indeed doubling up as an X-ray machine. The unawareness, illiteracy and gullibility of the people were eating up the insides of the society.

The quacks were ominous as they pretended to be doctors and treaded paths where real doctors would fear to go. Most countries have quacks but the percentage in Kapashera was one doctor to a hundred quacks. They would undertake all kinds of treatments and prescribe wrong medications with wrong dosages. Most of the quacks gave medicines that were wrapped in bits of newspaper and contained a melange of coloured tablets which I learnt to identify as a painkiller, a steroid and a vitamin. The origin of these tablets was dubious. Not one of those medicines had the correct dosage. This cocktail of coloured tablets ensured that the fever came down. The patient would feel better but was never completely treated for the sickness. They became patients forever!

The diet restrictions the quacks placed would make the patient sicker. If it was jaundice, all yellow foods were banned. The simple minds of the villagers accepted this simple diktat. A new mother was forbidden any 'cold' foods which meant she was off all vegetables, fruits and salads, milk and yogurts. She could have only wheat porridge and boiled water. Since bathing was forbidden for a new mother, she would come wrapped up in blankets, looking frail, sick and wretched in the blistering heat of June and July. The mothers were housed in dark rooms with no light for at least two months as it was believed that it was the sun that caused infections. Sickness was thrust on them. Gradually, I drummed into them the healthy practices of a daily bath, the importance of green vegetables and lentils and, of course, the benefits of sunlight. Today, my heart feels happy when I see mothers looking happy and healthy as they come with their week-old babies. A lot has changed; maybe the pebble I flung in the water to create some whorls of change went too far. This learning is not taught in medical schools. It's a deep and slow learning and does not come from a superficial and dispassionate appraisal.

The sheer number of chronic typhoid cases I was seeing was not normal. With perpetual low doses that were being administered by the quacks, it was natural that the disease stayed in the bodies and the patient became a chronic typhoid carrier. They, in turn, infected many more. The patients kept suffering from low-grade fever for months on end. Many patients with a history of upset tummies, loss of appetite and weight loss would find their way into my clinic. Blood tests proved that my suspicions were correct. Most were invariably suffering from chronic typhoid. Once they received the proper dosage for the right duration, they were fine. Treating them properly and making them fit was not profitable for the quacks. What could be better for them than having a sick population? A GP has to run a comprehensive community health centre with the frugal resources available along with a sense of ethical responsibility.

There were many cases of prolonged fever who would stagger their way to my clinic. They would be breathless and emaciated, yet their faces would look roundish. Moon-faced, sickly and feverish, yet the fever was unrecordable. The gauntness that accompanies loss of weight was simply missing. Upon auscultation, I would find crackles and signs of pneumonia. Initially, I was a bit confused due to the absence of fever. On taking the detailed history, I would find that the patients were on high doses of steroids given by the quacks. Steroids that doctors use with utmost prudence were prescribed freely to all patients. They were cheap, they acted fast and they gave the patient a feeling of well-being. The signs of infection would be camouflaged while the infection kept flaring inside like a conflagration and manifested itself months later in deadly forms. Most of them were Tubercular. Some developed hydrothorax (fluid in the lungs) while others had cavities with fibrous walls around them, which were impossible to treat.

Some patients even had complete collapse of the lungs and succumbed to their disease. Some came in with the diagnosis proclaimed by the quack. "The blood has turned to water," in cases of jaundice or severe anaemia, or "the blood has become yellow," or 'blue" in cases of heart disease or choking where the child's fingers would turn blue. All these sound amusing but needed a lot of convincing over years and decades. If there had been no intervention by the quacks, thousands of patients would be alive today.

Abscesses and wounds were another dubious forte of the quacks. They would deal with these by putting some sticky substance and covering it with a leaf. The leaf would be secured with an old rag. The patient was instructed not to open it for ten to twelve days. I came across hundreds of these wounds—breast abscesses, abscesses caused by diabetes, infected wounds, all came to me but a bit too late. The patients came in with chills and rigors accompanied by a high fever due to the infection. Some abscesses could be treated in the clinic. Just to clean up the dubious, sticky pastes that the village quacks applied to the wound took hours. There were some abscesses that I could drain and some that had too much degeneration of tissue causing wounds as deep as craters. Appropriate antibiotics and dressings that were redone every day did help most of the patients. It was very frustrating to see patients with wounds that could have healed in a few days, coming in so late that they were beyond any hope. They went into full-blown septicaemia when the infection flowed through the bloodstream. Septicaemia can turn fatal very quickly. These patients had to be referred to Safdarjung Hospital (SFJ).

I know of one woman who had been going to a quack for

a foot abscess. He kept on applying some paste and tying it up with a leaf. When she finally came to me, I discovered that she had diabetes and the wound had eaten up her flesh and bored into the bone. I tried to treat her with antibiotics and daily dressings. When nothing helped, I referred her to SFJ hospital and later I heard that she had to have an amputation. She was only forty-five. These were many moments of helplessness and frustration that seemed to envelope me in a sense of failure.

Renal and gall bladder stones were another lucrative business for these quacks. These invincible men would keep some multi-coloured powders in small glass jars. Probably they were taken from roadside trees and powdered. These powders were dispensed wrapped in bits of newspaper. The gullible patients took them happily in the hope of getting rid of the stones. The medicines weren't cheap. The quacks prescribed them for months and laughed all the way to the bank. When the patients went back after a couple of months for a check-up, the crook would go into his dark dingy hole and come out with one or two stones on his palm. He would show the stones to the patient, "Look, your stones fell out of your gall bladder into my room." The naive patient would go home relieved that he had been rid of his kidney stones.

There were cases of asthmatic bronchitis who were desperate for any treatment that would cure them. Whenever a disease is chronic, the role of the quacks becomes inextricably important. I knew of some Babas who would put some ash onto the patient's tongue or forehead. Lo and behold, the patients would be cured of their asthma. Was the sickness and its treatment all in the mind? I wondered many times!

Hundreds of fascinating stories found their way into my

clinic. Like little spores, they germinated and occupied spaces in my mind clogging it. There was this Baba who would make the patient swallow a small fish that was guaranteed to make the asthma disappear, or so I heard. This Baba had serpentine queues outside his little shanty. People travelled from all over the country for that little fish to be placed on their tongues. The folklores, the incredible stories of complete cure, all added to a stupendous faith. I am sure a lot of people were cured of their asthma for faith is the strongest healer. I shouldn't criticise these quacks for I was dispensing placebos too. With my medical knowledge, I knew where to draw the line so as not to harm the patient and knew when to stop and let them go to a tertiary care facility. With every fish-eating patient who got cured, there were thousands who died believing their asthma was cured and refused to ask for medical help. Patients brought in by wives, sons and daughters, who could barely pull in a breath, would refuse all medicines. "The Baba gave me a magic fish so nothing can happen to me." Seeing them collapse in my waiting room was sad.

Certain unethical and illiterate quacks dared to perform surgeries too. They were doing termination of pregnancies, appendectomies and hernias. I do not know how they managed without anaesthesia. I learnt of their surgical prowess from a number of patients who had had their appendixes removed by Dr Biswas. On an ultrasound, the patient's appendix was intact. I presume that they were just making a shallow incision and stitching it up so the scar was real and no one knew if they still had an appendix or not. I heard of many cases where they would leave patients bleeding on the table and scoot off to set up practice in another hole in another hamlet under another name. It would be heard in the village the next morning that "Ram Kumar's wife died yesterday."

"How did she die?" I quizzed Ram Kumar's neighbour.

"Oh she had a pain in her stomach and went to the local doctor; must be some curse". They just accepted it as God's curse which explained everything that could not be explained by logic or science. The quacks got away easily all the time.

Was it the acceptance of hopelessness or helplessness?

The dais have been, and still are, the backbone of the childbirth processes in India. They are the local women who help in childbirth at home. They are not trained but after conducting so many home births they become formidable authorities on childbirth. They fulfil the great vacuum created by a lack of doctors in remote villages. They can manage standard deliveries easily. Transverse or Breech deliveries are difficult, but I have seen them conduct these successfully as well. One in a hundred may go wrong, but that happens in the best medical centres, too. I never resented the dais. They asked for very little payment and most times, a bag of rice or a saree sufficed.

What was scary were the foreign objects they inserted in the vagina for various ailments. Sometimes, stories of these self-appointed "sex experts" would outright turn into horror stories. I once had a female patient who came in with severe pain in the abdomen. On an internal examination, I felt something unfamiliar. I withdrew it with forceps. It was a glass bangle that had been inserted in her vagina. "What is this?" I asked the patient, horrified.

"I had a bit of looseness in my vagina, so the dai inserted this bangle," she said promptly. I was aghast.

"When was this?" I tried to moderate the alarm in my tone.

"Oh, maybe two or three years back."

The bangle was severely infected, and foul-smelling. A putrid collection of pus had collected around it and had been causing her pain. Later during my practice, I came across various kinds of treatments for loosened vaginas, or even third degree prolapse of the uterus which caused the entire uterus to hang outside the perineum. Uterine prolapses were very common because most of the child births were conducted at home either by the mothers-in-law or the dais. There was no concept of an episiotomy to reduce the pull on the uterus. The final goal was to take the baby out. No one bothered about the mother. Hence, women in their twenties lived lives of indignity and shame with prolapse of the uterus and unforgivable tears of the vagina causing incontinence of urine. And they lived with it. With no recourse to any good clinics the only solutions were mechanical. Leather rings and clay bangles were inserted inside the vaginas to stop the uterus from hanging outside.

There were other reasons to insert interesting objects in the vaginas. Over the years, I discovered many such objects in this part of the anatomy. Pieces of wood, a small candle and even a strip of leather. I have withdrawn these objects in my clinic. I learnt that these were inserted either for fertility or contraception and sometimes to increase her libido.

The village women were excellent storytellers. All they needed was a good ear which I provided because my need to understand these people was great and urgent. I heard hundreds of strange stories about life in villages. An example was the gender discrimination that made life a living hell for most women. When on a train, one must have seen the advertisements of sex specialists who assure the men of unending manly powers and strength, plastered on the walls. Phone numbers of these sex experts are printed in large letters. I have never seen these kinds of advertisements in any other country I have been to. Maybe men in India need some extra strength. Or maybe, indoctrination across generations and popular Indian culture had taught them that the sole purpose of their lives was to become the ultimate macho man through virility and endless physical strength, and the display of that in bed.

My woes appeared very petty in comparison to these women's. I discovered that this colossal population had no recourse to any legitimate medical guidance at all. Naturally, ignorance had to give rise to fear. Fear leads to illogical behaviours and development of blind faith in the unknown. The quacks were cashing in on these fears. In my early years, I would be caught off guard if a patient said, "My wife is cold." Or when a female patient complained saying, "My husband doesn't satisfy me." These issues have come into the limelight almost three decades later in the urban world. I dealt with them in the eighties because I kept an open ear for these simple villagers. The placebos came to my rescue in treating these unfamiliar ailments. I handed out placebos with utmost earnestness and a prayer on my lips. There was nothing else I could do to treat these diseases of the mind. If I didn't give the patient a big packet of multi-coloured tablets, I knew they would visit a quack and receive dubious cocktails. Feeling guilty, I patted myself when most of the men came back asking for more of my multivitamin packets.

"Your medicines were very good," a beaming Saryu would say. "Give me more of those." Placebos acquired a very high place of respect in my medical repertoire and I can recount hundreds of more tales extolling their benefits.

Chickenpox, measles and mumps were all believed to be caused by a Goddess. When people believe that a disease has no cure and that it comes and goes on its own, it has to be caused by a God or Goddess. Even today, it is no mean task to convince them otherwise. I yield to their beliefs and tell them that it will take its course as long as we can prevent complications. Voodoo is still a treatment of choice for all viral infections and even typhoid and jaundice. Mental illnesses were believed to be caused by spirits. "The spirit has entered her body, I have to take her to the Baba for *Jhara*," said Shrimati, one of my regular patients. Her daughter had stopped eating and would just stare into space.

People took the patient to the Voodoo guy who ran a broom over them to cleanse them of the curse of the Goddess. As long as they did not take any medication from the Voodoo guy, I had no problem.

One of them, Shatru Singh, was a very popular Voodoo guy who was believed to treat all kinds of typhoid and jaundice patients. A lot of my patients would go to him. The queues outside his shanty were legendary. Once, when one of my patients suffering from jaundice insisted on visiting this Voodoo guy, I convinced him to give me a bit of the medicine for analysis. I sent those medicines for testing in a laboratory and sure enough, they all contained steroids in very high doses. No amount of coaxing and reasoning convinced the patients that he was a hoax. There was hope and honour in the Voodoo guys as they never pretended to be doctors like the quacks. The voodoo treatment was usually limited to the broomstick, incense and applying ash on the body. It wasn't harmful even if the sickness wasn't cured.

There were certain times when it did cure; I presumed it must be due to the placebo effects of the broom and the fanfare.

Another variety of treatment centres were of the Babas, the religious sadhus. They had a blind following. A fascinating case of a young woman called Usha was one that one reads about only in books. She was the victim of one of the biggest yet commonest frauds occurring in India. I had read about it in my obstetrics book. A term called pseudo pregnancy. It was an unimportant entity in our medical books and was without much relevance in the examinations. It was just a one-liner definition in the book of Obstetrics and Gynaecology. I remember we had all laughed at it in the final year. How was it possible to fake a pregnancy? Little did I know that it was a real psychosomatic illness.

Usha came to me accompanied by her mother-in-law, sister-in-law, sister-in-law's husband and her husband. They had hired a tractor from Bahadurgarh to come to my clinic. They all had this air of expectancy and urgency, which I gathered was because the stakes were high. Usha was clearly pregnant; she looked full term. She waddled into my clinic in the typical lordosis posture of pregnancy and the family stared at me in silence. "Can you please check her?" said the mother-in-law. "Just see if the baby is okay." I lay her down on the examination bench and felt her abdomen. It was big all right, but I could not feel the baby's head and limbs. I used the Doppler but could not hear any heartbeats.

"Let's get an ultrasound done," I said finally before voicing my fears.

"Oh we can't," three voices said in unison. They all cast furtive glances at each other as if they were all party to some conspiracy.

Looking at them, a bit confused and irritated, I said, "Why not?"

"The Baba told us not to get an ultrasound done till she delivers the baby," said the husband. Since he looked the most amenable, I addressed him, shunning the others and said, "If we do the ultrasound and the baby is weak, I can give some medicines. If you don't get the ultrasound, I will not be able to help you," I said gently, still looking at the husband.

He seemed to agree. They all went out and huddled in a conference in hushed whispers.

"Ok, we will get it done," announced the husband.

When the family came back with the ultrasound report, I was surprised.

There was no pregnancy at all. I had suspected it but had left a space of doubt in my suspicion. This was a typical case of pseudo pregnancy.

The woman had been convinced by the Baba that she was pregnant. The strength of the mind and the belief that she was pregnant played havoc with her hormones. Her periods stopped. As with most pregnant women, she had let loose her abdomen so that it looked big and pregnant. Such is the power of the mind. Many questions haunted my scientific mind.

How did she miss her periods for so long?

How did her abdomen grow so large? How did the family believe that she was pregnant for nine months?

How, how, and how?

I knew the scientific knowledge we have is just the tip of the iceberg.

The cunning Baba had told them never to go to a doctor and not get an ultrasound done. I came across many such

Baba-induced pregnancies later. These Babas were like the voodoo guys but passed off as direct agents of God. The family, especially the mother-in-law who desperately wanted an heir, was a disconsolate wreck and started to sob. I learnt that they had paid lakhs of rupees to Baba.

Not being able to produce a child is anathema in this prolific society where a man's worth and success is measured by the number of children he can bear, yet, there is no way a man can be responsible for infertility. It is the sole curse of the woman to bear. A barren woman was discarded in favour of a new bride. This practice had the sanction of the society. Even when confronted with reports that showed zero sperm counts, the men would never believe the news.

When dealing with infertility cases, I came across some cases that would find their way into imaginative fiction. There were many men with zero sperm counts probably because of having mumps in childhood. It's a well-known fact that mumps can affect the production of sperms by the testes. Since the mumps vaccine was not on the mandatory list of the government till a few years back, there were a large number of men with a zero sperm count. Once I diagnosed a man with a nil sperm count he would never come back to continue the treatment for he could not bear to accept the fact of being the cause of childlessness. They believed that infertility was the woman's curse. A few did come back a year later with a baby in their arms.

"How come, Sheela?" I asked the new mother.

"Oh, we went to a Baba," Sheela would bend her head down coyly and say softly.

"But your husband has no sperm," I would persist in my ignorance.

"Baba can do everything," came the pat reply from a joyous Sheela who refused to meet my eyes.

Later, when I was not so ignorant, I learnt that the Baba would take the childless women into his chambers and give them the precious gift of a baby. The mother-in-law paid the donation which was more of a service fee. The whole family knew about the deal. The young wife knew but the family kept this a secret from the husband. It was a convenient arrangement. The infertile woman would get pregnant and neighbours and relatives would stop hounding her for being barren. With a baby in her arms, she would not be thrown out of the husband's home for not bearing a child.

The worst and most worrying part is that these quacks and the Voodoo guys still thrive and the villagers still believe in them. I have to compete with their non-existent knowledge and their frenetic following. I genuinely believe that child mortality and sickness levels will fall drastically if the government flushes out these killer, fake doctors. The end of the nineties brought in some pleasant changes. There were more hospital deliveries. The dais were given incentives by the government to get expectant mothers to the hospital. They were paid to administer the mandatory tetanus shots and distribute iron and folic acid tablets. It worked well for all.

CHAPTER EIGHT

Bijwasan

BIJWASAN WAS ABOUT a twenty-minute walk from my clinic. I had never set foot in the village of Bijwasan, yet I could picture it from the details my patients gave me. I knew the people were affluent compared to others from their attire, gait and the nicely-painted tractors they arrived in. Some of them owned large acres of land and sprawling homes and lived in large, joint families headed by great-grandparents. One could presume that sickness was scarce and longevity was the rule. It was not difficult to surmise that they lived an idyllic existence with plentitude. There are some places that are blessed with warm sunlight, abundant crops, beautiful people and generous families. Bijwasan was one of those.

It was all of this and more. The people of this village were different from the other villagers. They had wonderful genes. The women with aquiline noses, towered high above the others, as they ambled in elegantly with their stately postures. They were fair by Indian standards and some even had greyish-blue eyes. The men had a good ruddy complexion and were handsome with chiselled features. A lot of male models on the Indian ramp were from this area. Wrestling was a favourite pastime in Bijwasan. A few wrestlers made it to the Indian Olympic team. I cherished and enjoyed looking at these comely faces as they walked into my clinic; each pretty face was a story in itself and a delightful sight.

At times, women brought their blue-eyed babies into the clinic and I would find it difficult to take my eyes away from such beauty. I often wondered about the source of those fantastic genes. Some of them were so pretty that I could only stare and speculate about the stir these women would cause on the fashion scene. The most endearing part about them was that they were blissfully unaware of their stunning looks. These women were not allowed to work outside of their homes, so the world missed out on their unparalleled beauty that filled me with awe.

I knew that these folks had taken a fancy to me and came in hordes. The fancy was mutual as I loved to talk, treat and teach them. Some came with their woes and others came just to gape at me. A visit to my clinic was an excuse for a social outing and the waiting room became a social club for the villagers to meet and greet each other and natter about their work, families and their crops. They gathered in my clinic for a chat which at most times did not involve a medical consultation.

Most private clinics and larger public hospitals would never encourage people clubbing in the waiting room and would find it irksome. But I loved the camaraderie and the family scenes in my waiting room. I marvelled at the simple laughter and happiness that emanated from these crowds. They sat in family groups, at times with their legs folded comfortably under them, faces illumined with love.

It especially warmed my heart when my waiting room became a rendezvous to invite and meet married daughters who resided in far-off villages. There were unwritten but firm rules in place for married girls. They could not visit the parental home without the permission of the mother-in-law. At times years went by without a visit to her parents. Ironically, they were allowed to visit my clinic as a visit to the doctor raised no eyebrows. Also, no mother-in-law wanted a sick workhorse. The moment the mother heard that her daughter was visiting me, the whole maternal gang would come right in the morning and camp in my waiting room till the dear daughter arrived. The joy in the girl's eyes when she saw her brothers, her father and her old mother and a few neighbours, was unparalleled. My eyes would turn a wee bit misty as I saw the entire maternal gang looking at her with loving and longing eyes. The mother would feed her the bajra rotis smeared with ghee and laddoos she had got for her. The father would pour the fresh buttermilk in clay cups from the gallons he carried in the tractor. A happy family, sitting with cups of buttermilk, sipping and talking, murmuring sweet nothings, filled my clinic with joy.

Just being instrumental in getting a family together and being a tiny part of that joy made my job worthwhile.

Almost all clinics have that sickly, antiseptic smell that overwhelms the senses and pervades the waiting rooms, examination rooms and the couches that stand there. My clinic had a different smell. It smelled of spices and onions and pickles on most days. It smelled of home, love and buttermilk. Soon mobile street food vendors set up shop outside the clinic.

They sold fast food and snacks. I could inhale the aromas of samosas and bread pakoras from my waiting room. They were doing brisk business. I knew the clinic was spreading happiness in its own way, treating the body and the heart. Wasn't this my father's vision?

After their fill of spicy food, it was natural that the patients became somniferous. They put their legs up and dozed off by the cool air of the water cooler. Why would I mind that? It was the smell and sight of rapt contentment. If I could provide a sanguine and safe place for a few people, it was enough for me.

It made more sense for the Bijwasan folks to bring everyone along as the trailer could hold about thirty people. A single visit to my clinic became a grand festive affair as well as a family outing. The grandmothers, in-laws, wives, cousins and even the neighbours would sit in the back of the family tractor, clad in their best lehengas and *odhnis*. Not all were patients, of course. If one tractor load got cured, I would see another load of thirty patients the very next day. These families, in turn, would sing praises of the new, young doctor who always wore sarees. It was only a matter of time before entire villages adopted me as their 'family doctor'. They would walk into my clinic smiling as if I was their long-lost friend. We exchanged pleasantries about each other's families. They would keep track of my children; I would inquire about theirs, their ageing mothers, their cattle and their yield of wheat.

It was these patients who reverently filed into the clinic with their deep faith and optimistic belief in me, that helped me survive those years of utter despair and desolation. I saw piquant family scenes, heard strange stories, learnt their dialects, their mores and celebrated their joys and mourned their losses.

Although the patients provided exciting challenges for me, I knew I was playing with fire. It was the will of the Gods that I survived unscathed as the blood ran passionately in Bijwasan. They were more genial and sociable than others on good days but could spit vengeance if stoked and dire consequences could follow. There was a family from Bijwasan who became one of my most regular patients. It was a large joint family. There were four brothers with three children each. The parents, too, lived with the sons in the large house. My first encounter with the family was when one of the sons came to me and said, "We all will come to you from today." His words sounded like a grave verdict.

"Why me?" I asked in the same grave tone.

"The doctor we were going to in Bijwasan gave a wrong injection to my son," he said, a bit agitated.

"My son died," he said softly. He paused and looked around to see if anyone was within earshot. Then he bent lower so he could whisper in my ear, "We pulled her out of her clinic and beat her up."

This made me look up and take a long look at him. A hundred thoughts crossed my mind. It could happen to me. Did I really want to treat anyone from this family?

"My clinic is very small," I started to say. "I don't have all the facilities. It will be better if you take the children to a specialist." I tried to dissuade him.

"No, we will come to you," he said resolutely.

Just as the patients can choose their doctors, I wish doctors could choose their patients too. It was not fair; I felt duty bound. I had to relent. There was no arguing or reasoning with the Bijwasan folks. These kind of people were fraught with the risk of violence in the future. Well, I did treat all the children of this family for years but with trepidation. The children have grown into tall, strapping lads and girls. Some have joined the army while others have taken up modelling. The girls have gotten married in respectable homes. One of the young men, I heard, participated in the Olympics as part of the Indian wrestling team. A few did MBA and went where their jobs took them. Even if they relocated to other cities, their Delhi visits always include a visit to me. They walk in with pleasant faces, just to make sure I am alive and healthy. At times it feels that these children are my numerous trophies. It makes me happy when these boys bring their own children for treatment. It was a miracle I survived unscathed.

I made many long-term relationships with these villagers which continues to this day.

"I haven't seen Savitri for a long time," I would say to my staff as Savitri brought with her laughter and a blitheness that I needed. Like a wish fulfilled, I would see Savitri walk in smiling affectionately at me. As I said before, I was preordained to be a part of these people. It could not have been otherwise. Another favourite of mine was a matriarch Sharbati who still visits me because she has high cholesterol and a renal stone. She came in a few years back, a picture of bliss. "Look, my grandson," she held the baby and removed the white towel from the face so I could get a good look at him.

"Very nice baby, so pretty," I said naturally. "What have you named him?"

"Balesh," came the prompt, proud reply. To say I was taken aback would be an understatement. This was the first baby I came across who was my namesake. Little did I know that many more would follow later.

"It's the best name," said the grandmother happily. "I hope he becomes a doctor like you." She beamed at the baby and the baby beamed at me. "Even my neighbour has named her daughter Balesh." I didn't have a copyright to my name. Now, twenty years later, Balesh is a handsome lad of twenty. He bought a fleet of cars with the money he received from the sale of the farmland, and rented them out. He is all of twenty and his parents are looking for a suitable match for him.

Bijwasan was inseparable from my practice as the majority of my patients hailed from this prosperous village. It had a very dark side too which I discovered down the line. The railway track was one of the dark spots in the prosperity of Bijwasan which I will mention later.

A handful of the young men who were my patients chose to opt for world-class wrestling or modelling. In the nineties, when awareness struck, some of them joined the new genre of gyms and became enthusiastic gym clients. They visited the clinic for consultations about their diet to build muscle and stamina. At times, they came with injuries due to over exercising. When one of the young lads, Monu, got selected for the Indian wrestling team, big, noisy celebrations happened. He was taken around in a tractor decorated with flowers and balloons with the loudspeakers blaring Bollywood songs. He came to the clinic with a big box of sweets. "This is for you Ma'am," he said shyly, still wearing his marigold garland.

This event set the trend for the rest of the village boys to enroll for wrestling classes. Increased demand led to an increase in supply and hundreds of gyms opened shop. In no time, almost every house had a gym. Some of them were fly-by-night operators. They promised the moon, using every trick to build up muscle, leaving nothing to chance. Just a glance at a couple of these boys with their unnaturally rippling muscles and I knew I had to dig deeper for the cause. It turned out to be exactly what I had suspected. The gym owners were making quick bucks from these unsuspecting young guys and injecting them with hormones to build muscle. They were using the same syringes for many different people and they didn't care about the side effects. After all, it was all about the money. High protein powders of dubious contents, injections to build massive muscle and bone-breaking exercise routines were prescribed by the gym owners. They were untrained, illiterate village men who doubled up as gym instructors. The ambitious and naive boys were taken in by their false promises.

Very soon, the unethical protein concoctions and injections took their toll and it was visible to even untrained eyes. Young men would amble into my waiting room rippling with muscles, complaining of tiredness and joint pains. The worst were the injection abscesses. These abscesses were a new entrant to the repertoire of uncommon diseases I had witnessed. One of the young men, Sargam, an aspiring weightlifter, came to me with a very deep abscess. I discovered that he had received ten steroid injections. The abscess was deep and took almost two months to fill up. The steroid trend was dangerous, for the steroids puffed up the boys' bodies and lowered the immunity which led to abscesses, fevers, tiredness and loss of appetite.

This young man understood what the fake gym owners had done to him and started a movement to increase awareness. He started to talk to the village lads and convinced them about the pitfalls of taking steroid injections. Hundreds of boys were saved by his relentless campaign.

Alongside Sargam's campaign I, too, started warning these youngsters about the dangers of the steroids and powders that were handed out in the gyms. However, they still wanted to become wrestlers and models, so I gave them certified protein powders which kept them safe from the harmful ones and counselled them about how high protein and balanced diets worked in most cases. The young guys were driven and had just one goal…to be selected for the Indian wrestling or weightlifting team. Gradually, as these youngsters realised the harm that these injections could cause, they stopped falling into the trap, and the phony gyms started to close down.

Along with developing a healthy doctor-patient relationship with these young boys, I also built a bond with the rest of the young population. Unlike their parents who were not aware of changing times and still lived in the past, I related to their problems and displayed a more profound understanding. Some parents did not accept the changes of the modern world, so their children were left with limited guidance and support. The children were watching endless television channels and were exposed to the modern world. Their aspirations and ambitions were changing fast.

A young man called Shailesh, who had been selected for the CRPF (Central Reserve Police Force), was one I was fond of as he was hardworking and had heeded my advice to take control of his life. It was tough to gain admission in this reputed institution because the entry requirements were extremely stringent. Very few young men found themselves on the admission list. Shailesh was sent to their training centre which was a few hundred kilometres away from Kapashera.

"My poor son has to go so far," wailed his anguished mother. "He has eaten only home cooked meals," she went on. No amount of wailing could help her as the physical training was mandatory.

One regular afternoon as I tried to finish the daily influx of patients, a tall, affable looking young man, in a khaki uniform, walked in. My staff followed him a bit piqued as he had not taken the queue number. He walked straight to my desk with a huge smile. The young lad looked fetching in his police uniform. Of course, that was Shailesh.

"Good morning, Doctor," he said with an unfamiliar confidence.

"Hello Sonu," I addressed him by his pet name that I had used since he was a toddler. "What happened?"

His smile vanished and he looked a little distraught and agitated. "I have run away from the academy."

"Does your mother know?" I asked.

"No, she does not." Shailesh paused to look at my reaction. "I came straight to you," he continued. "She might get upset."

"Why did you run away?"

"Look," he said as he took off his shoes and socks and lifted one foot over the other leg so I could get a better view. To my dismay, his entire sole was ulcerated and oozing fluid.

I exclaimed, "Let me see what I can do, but do call your mother."

He called his mother who lived nearby in Bijwasan.

"How did it happen?" I asked.

"They give us thin-soled shoes and make us run ten miles every day in the blazing heat," he complained, sure that he would receive some sympathy.

As Shailesh completed his sentence, I sensed that all he needed and had come for were some words of kindness and sympathy. After all, he was only eighteen and had stepped into the real world too soon. The ulcers were superficial and caused by heat and pressure. I knew they would heal in three to four days. I felt terrible for him as I knew the training was gruelling. Since it was mandatory, he had to complete his time and there was no way that he could leave.

Soon his mother arrived, panting, breathless and worried.

"My son, my poor son," she fawned over her little boy. "What have they done to you?"

I watched his mother's reaction and knew I would have done the same for my son.

"It's okay, the ulcers are superficial and will heal in a few days," I declared. "I will give him a medical certificate for some leave."

"I am not going back there," said the boy petulantly.

"You must go back; it's important that you don't leave midway," I encouraged. "The other boys would give anything to be in your place."

There was no way I would let him leave the academy. Leaving a prestigious career midway was the biggest mistake he could make. I had seen the other village boys while away their days smoking and drinking; I didn't want Shailesh to follow in their footsteps. The mother seemed to understand my concerns and she tried to drum some sense into him.

"I will write an application that you should get proper sports shoes for running." I hoped this solution would work and he would not lose his privileged spot. Three years later, Shailesh was enlisted as a permanent recruit into CRPF; he had got married and had one child. He never stopped thanking me whenever he came to the clinic with his infant.

Some of the women would walk long distances to the clinic just to tell me about a wedding in the family or the sickness of their cow. Emotional narratives about their mother-in-law's behaviour; their husband's sister's taunts and tearful stories of their husband's indifference—all enamoured me like a gripping script of a movie. The experiences were narrated amidst sobs and sniffles. Many people would likely have grown tired of hearing such things but not me.

"This year was good, we got two tonnes of wheat," Savitri would say with pride. The news of the bountiful monsoon reached me not from newspapers but from the farmers themselves. A bad monsoon meant a bad crop, and a bad crop meant less money for the whole year, which translated into fewer patients for me. Fewer patients meant that the villagers would neglect their medicines and not come up for routine check-ups. Their absence resulted in uncontrolled diabetes, low birth weights, missed vaccinations, increased alcohol consumption and malnutrition in children. In short, a bad crop meant that the whole wheel of diseases would unfurl and I could not help but notice these changes.

After examining and treating five generations over forty years, there are some dichotomies in my medical knowledge. I wonder why none of the chronic smokers that I badgered to stop smoking didn't die of cancer? I wonder why the alcoholics didn't die of liver failures? The men who guzzled bottles of whiskey still do so and I continue to see them perfectly happy as they plod along, content in their ignorance and their semi-alert state of mind. Their livers haven't packed up yet. I haven't seen the hookah smokers' lungs go into complete fibrosis. Furthermore, the chain smokers haven't developed lung carcinoma and I don't see any cardiac strokes from having full-fat buffalo milk and ladles of ghee.

I wonder how much truth is there in all of these warnings!

Since I have observed four to five generations of people, I can confidently say that I have lived through a massive linear study of disease patterns. However, these disease patterns do not follow the rules and progression of disease that we were taught in medical school, and they do not fall into the moulds of the fancy Harvard studies that enumerate the causative factors of cancer, liver disease, cardiac disease and many more.

CHAPTER NINE

My Clinic

ONE DAY IN the late afternoon, two men entered the clinic. One looked a bit weak and pale. During my time as a GP, I have learnt that there are many different kinds of pallor, and with enough experience one can distinguish the difference between the pallor of anaemia, renal failure, liver failure and a heart attack.

"What is the problem?" I asked.

"He was working in the office," the other man stuttered. "Then he vomited and felt weak."

One look at the man and I knew that I had to send him to the hospital.

"You need to take him to Safdarjung," I said in a definitive tone.

"Please, Doctor, just treat him here," pleaded the other man. "We can't take him anywhere as he lives very far away."

I reconsidered and thought as I negotiated the diagnosis in my mind.

It could be just plain vomiting.

As I was about to cave in, I examined his face. I knew in an instant that it was not plain vomiting due to the greyness of his skin. He had to be sent to the hospital and fast.

I took the other man aside and told him that I suspected a Myocardial Infarction or a heart attack.

"No, no, it's not possible," he panicked defensively. "He was fine just a moment ago."

"You need to take him quickly," I insisted.

The following day, he called to thank me and informed me that his friend had indeed suffered a heart attack and was saved because of my quick referral.

The distance between life and death is short. It's all about that one second. In that split second, one can judge wrongly and lose a patient. The moment someone sits in the consultation room at a small 4/4 feet table with a small letterhead, an inexpensive stethoscope, a steel torch and a small wooden stool, one is all alone. There are no senior residents to turn to if a patient stops breathing; no nurses to calculate the electrolytes that need to be pumped into a lifeless, limp body; and no one behind your shoulder as you witness an epileptic child frothing at the mouth and convulsing spasmodically. Regarding the latter, I would just give the correct dosage of Diazepam and wait and repeat if necessary, just as we were taught. Most of the time, the child would be relieved of the convulsions and the parents would look gratefully at me as they carried the sleepy child in their arms.

Once, there was a two-year-old child, Sonu, who had come a few times earlier for epileptic attacks. He lay helplessly on my examination bench as he convulsed and frothed with glassy eyes, but he always responded to my shots of Diazepam and I never had to repeat a shot for him. Even though I had prescribed the usual medicines for epilepsy that had to be taken, I suspected that the mother failed to be regular as he came in at least once in two months.

A couple of weeks later, the mother rushed in with the convulsing child in her arms.

"Quickly, lay him here," I said pointing to the table.

I gave my shot and waited for the muscles to relax. Five, six, seven, eight minutes went by and the convulsions were as strong as before. At ten minutes, I gave the second shot and waited again. One, two, three… I counted with bated breath… five, six and seven minutes went by. The child was stiff and still in a convulsive state. There was no sign of the body loosening. I knew the child had gone into Status Epilepticus.

My brain was working like a spinning machine. There was no help anywhere near. I realised the vulnerability of practising in this area; I could turn nowhere for help.

A new paediatrician had opened up shop just across the road. It was obvious that if I sent the mother to Safdarjung which was an hour away, it might be too late. I sensed that the mother's confidence in me had become rickety. "Why don't you try the new doctor across the road?" I looked at her impassive face and could not figure out her thought process. Without a word, she picked up her child and crossed the road to find the new paediatrician. Within five minutes she was back, her face tear stained. "He refused to see my child."

This rankled deep. I felt helpless. The new doctor should have seen the child and tried to help but I could understand his refusal. The child was my patient and he saw me as his competitor so it was natural he didn't want to step in at a late stage.

"You need to take him to Safdarjung, they will be able to help."

"How do I go there, I have no conveyance?" She rasped at me, clearly aggrieved.

"You need to take him there immediately." Even as I said this, I saw that the child suddenly had become flaccid. He wasn't taut anymore. I looked into his pupils, felt the pulse and saw the pallor almost all at once. The mother's face changed from one of grievance to accusation in a matter of seconds. Her beady eyes looked accusingly and aggressively at me.

I knew the battle for the life of the child was over.

But the battle of my life had just started.

"You've killed my child!" said the mother accusingly. She was inconsolable and pushed the glass of water away which my staff offered her. I was disconcerted and felt cornered.

"Please call your husband," I said gently.

"Hmmm, I will, surely I will."

I was shaken too, as it was the first death in my clinic in over two decades.

"If you had not given him the injection, my child would still be alive," she sobbed.

A dead patient and an accusing relative is the ultimate nightmare for all doctors.

There was no point in justifying myself or looking for absolution as she was in no condition to listen or reason. Her husband arrived ten minutes later. I told him that the child did not respond to the treatment and that it was common for that to happen. I expected to face his wrath, but the husband seemed to understand. "Yes, doctor, you are right, I am sure you did your best," he said. "It is God's will."

He took the child in his arms and walked away quietly.

Besides the crisis that ensued in my clinic that day, another battle awaited me at home. I had to recount the whole incident to my husband. I was certain that being the disciplinarian he was for medical protocols, he would find many faults in my line of action. After listening to my narrative in detail, he thought for a while and said, "It's not your fault."

I looked up in surprise and relief. He was my biggest litmus test.

"You did what any good doctor would have done."

I could have cried in the comforting solace his words gave me.

"I hope you realise that heroism does not work in real life," he reasoned patiently, "for along with the deification comes the risk of being attacked and vilified."

I heard his sombre words and vowed to be more selective in my patients. I stopped treating epilepsy patients and some emergencies after that day. The children with asthamatic bronchitis and epilepsy were the worst affected. I referred them all to SFJ with a heavy heart even though I knew that just one shot would cure them but I had to safeguard myself from serious implications. With that patient, I realised that along with immense glorification, denunciation is not far behind. No matter how adept I thought I was, I was defenseless in the face of unexpected accidents and the betrayal of the human body. Limitations of the art of medicine and the response of the human body to medicines had to be understood and respected. Along with the strategies for a private practice, I imbibed some survival techniques too.

My husband drilled into me the new and stricter guidelines that had been laid down for GPs over the years. Spontaneity, treating from the heart, trying to save the patients and other lofty ideals flew off like the years of youth that I had been clinging to.

Failures and loss of patients are the fastest teachers for a dilettante doctor.

A two-year-old child was brought to me once. The eyes looked glassy and unblinking. It appeared to be clearly dead on the first look. Instead of just shooing the mother away I thought that I would examine the baby as a show of empathy. There was no time or need to take a history of 'why', 'when', and 'how'? I asked the mother to lay him on the examination table. On auscultation, I could not hear even a whisper of a heartbeat. The stethoscope was silent as a rock. "No heroism," I remembered my husband's words. I should have sent the patient away, but I had to try something to revive the child, as my gut feeling said I could save the child. I tried CPR, but to no avail. The parents waited for a miracle, their eyes glued to my face. I looked at the parents and shook my head as words were not needed. The child had passed away. However, it wasn't that easy—the mother sobbed and pleaded for me to do something. "Please doctor, I have only one child," she wailed, "please help us, help us."

The evening at KWSCH in 1982 flashed before my eyes and I felt like a lone warrior who got left behind on the battlefield without her army. Suddenly, I felt a new determination and decided not to give up.

"Ok, I will try an injection," I said to the distressed mother. "It may help or it may not."

Following my gut feeling I remembered the evening in KWSCH where I had witnessed the same procedure in the ward. Armed with a syringe full of adrenaline, the magic drug, I thought awhile, doubting the sanity of my decision. I had promised my husband that there would be no more heroics and no more of trying to play God, yet I knew I had to try to save the child. My heart beat faster in anticipation and fear. I had never given an intracardiac injection alone, ever. There was no time to think and weigh; it had to be done. Holding the syringe steadily in my hand, I injected the adrenaline straight into the child's heart and continued the resuscitation. With all my prayers and belief, I waited and continued pumping the heart with my hands. The evening in KSCH had taught me the exact amount of pressure to apply to a child's heart without cracking the soft ribs.

Lo and behold! The child coughed and moved his legs. The mother, my staff of three girls and I looked at each other, speechless and incredulous. Patting the child's back to elicit more crying, I handed the child to the mother. She immediately pressed him to her chest. I realised that rare occasions such as this was the stuff of miracles. I also realised at that moment that it was some higher power that had brought the child back. It wasn't the injection, or the CRP. It was preordained that the child had to survive. I never repeated an intracardiac adrenaline injection as my husband warned me that these gallant acts could get me into grave trouble and I knew that he had a valid point. A private practice is a highly vulnerable place to be in because the GP doesn't have the backing of paramedical and other medical staff. Just one patient who may succumb can be a nemesis for any doctor.

Asthmatic children were more predictable in their response rate. A heavily wheezing child would settle down with regular breathing after a few minutes of the nebuliser, but many children lost their lives to asthma and epilepsy before my arrival on the scene. Gastroenteritis was another common cause of death. Mortality rate due to these big three dwindled to zero in just two or three years. It was not that I needed any special knowledge or powers to achieve this; it was just my presence in that area at the right time.

On taking a detailed history, I got to know that almost every family had lost an infant to either fever or gastroenteritis. I vowed to myself that I would make sure that no child died of gastroenteritis. I spent a lot of extra time with various mothers to educate them about the benefits of oral solutions. For them, it was just water and they did not understand the importance of giving 'just' water.

In the summer months, hundreds of limp children came to my clinic with sunken eyes and fontanelles. They were so limp that it seemed hopeless to even try to revive them. They hadn't passed urine in hours and they would be vomiting with incessant stools, which was enough for a one-year-old to be suspended between life and death. Just prescribing some medicines and sending those children home never served any purpose. I asked the mothers to wait in the waiting room and the staff girls handed a glass of water with ORS to each one of them. The mother would be closely monitored for putting spoonfuls of water in the little mouth. I would not allow them to leave until the child had passed urine. I employed an extra girl just to keep a watch on the restless mothers. At times, the exhausted mother would doze off but she had to be woken up to administer the life-saving fluid to her child. At times they had to sit for hours, but as soon as the child passed urine, the mother would be beaming. The change in the limp and lifeless child was magical. To see the child raise its head and look around was a joy few can experience.

The mothers resisted this exercise as they thought that sitting in the clinic just to give the child water was a waste of time. Some were in a hurry to get back and make lunch for the rest of the family. After a while, they realised that this was non-negotiable and that the results were fruitful. After hundreds of these children got treated, word got around that this corner clinic was the best for gastroenteritis.

All this water giving and monitoring turned my clinic into a daycare centre, which lengthened my working hours. I had to be around if a child did not pass urine or the fever did not come down. It was imperative that I stay back and decide whether to refer the child to Safdarjung in case the child didn't improve. Those decisions meant life or death for the patient as well as for me. If I failed to refer a child to the hospital at the right time, the entire village would be baying for my blood. Even though my confidence soared with these successes, I had a lot of learning to do. I realised that we were taught a fraction of what I really needed to know in a real practice, especially a rural one.

If things didn't go the right way, most patients accepted the verdict of death very calmly. I found their acceptance of death very repulsive for losing a child involved a short period of grieving until the woman became pregnant again. The dead child was soon forgotten. I saw that this resilience for death was common and came easily to these villagers. It appalled me to see so much complacency about sickness and death.

I saw all kinds of sick children in my clinic. Thanks to the thousands of children that I dealt with in KSCH, I could calculate and prescribe the correct dosage of the correct drug so they didn't have too much or too little. This was unheard of in Kapashera where the quacks were giving concoctions of ten different antibiotics but never enough of one. As a result, before my arrival on the scene, the children in Kapashera and all the numerous satellite hamlets were perpetually sick, malnourished, irritable and prone to dying. This was good business for the quacks. I took it as a personal challenge to change this. As they started to come to me, if one child recovered with the correct dosage, ten more would find their way to my clinic.

Soon enough, word got around about the doctor who could make your child healthy. Their underweight frames had been dosed with ineffective medicines or overdosed with antibiotics. The fevers were kept down even as the infections burnt inside. They would come so late to me that at times to revive life was barely a viable option.

Gradually I set to work on these children. Convincing the mothers of the importance of completing the full course of antibiotics proved to be a major task. Chiding the mothers if they missed doses or missed a visit to the clinic for follow-up was frustrating but worked in the long run. Almost all my child patients took just one antibiotic for years. I never gave them the second line of antibiotics but kept them in reserve. It took years for the patients to accept that I would not change the medicines every two days just to please them. They asked for different medicines at every visit. I would give the same one but would change the company and the colour. Most of my children grew up to be adults with just one antibiotic and never developed resistance to any antibiotic. As awareness increased, mothers started observing and appreciating this fact.

The benefits of my treatment did not take long to show as children are like flowers—quick to wither and quick to revive with good care. The children who visited me regularly looked much healthier with fewer episodes of sickness.

The cases of pneumonia, typhoid and malnutrition fell drastically in my catchment area. These mothers became my ambassadors and soon, a lot of children from the various hamlets, no matter how remote, crowded my waiting room. They had sunken eyes, bloated tummies, skinny legs and dull expressions. Some were grossly malnourished and had perpetually runny noses or diarrhoea.

Regular treatment and a good diet later, they looked bright and healthy. Furthermore, supplements of iron and protein and a bag full of good advice, worked wonders.

Their immunity levels went up and their mothers' confidence soared.

On the day of the clinic visit, the mothers would bathe them, and dress them proudly in washed and ironed clothes because they knew I would compliment them. Their labour never went in vain. I praised them within hearing of the other mothers present in the clinic. The praise and adulation had a snowball effect in the village.

"Oh, Sonu looks so good today. His shirt is so nice and clean," I would proclaim loud and clear so all patients would look at the beaming mom. This was like a personal trophy for these women. The next day a few other moms would dress up their child. What did it cost me? A few minutes of my time.

On the next visit, the mother would make extra effort to

wear better clothes herself, and soon, it became a joyful cycle of praise and acknowledgement for all of us.

In just a few years, anyone could notice that 'my children' looked noticeably different from the other kids in the village. They were all vaccinated with DPT, BCG, and measles. They were safe even when the whole village was stricken with measles or mumps. Most mothers thought that a consultation fee was a superfluous entity, but that notion changed over the years.

A baby-weighing machine was the single investment that paid off rich dividends. When the mothers saw the continuous weight gain of the little ones, they were reassured and went home happy. It was always the busiest corner of the clinic... the corner where the baby-weighing machine lay! It became a status symbol to be my patient, and they considered themselves lucky to have me in their lives.

Touching so many lives in such a positive way is what sustained me through my youth, middle age and now the sixties. The relatives who visited these mothers were always envious, so they brought their own children to me to ask me to wave a magic wand so their babies become just as healthy. There are many of them who still visit me for their grandchildren.

I was always ridden with self-doubt, regrets and even embarrassment at my choice of career, but today I feel that I was lucky to have Father, who had this great vision for me and believed I could do it. I know if I had worked in a fancy hospital, whether in India or abroad, I would not have touched even a small percentage of the lives I did here in Kapashera. I would have been just a rung of the well-oiled machinery and would have followed protocols and rules. Here, I made my own rules, broke my own rules and practised on my terms.

Snake bites, monkey bites, rat bites and even lizard bites were common cases I came across in the clinic. The number of snake bite cases were substantial as Kapashera had lots of large farmlands and forest cover in the eighties and nineties. As habitation increased, the reptiles moved around looking for new abodes. There were even cobra sightings. "It was this long, I know it was a cobra," said the lanky lad, his eyes dilated in fear. His uncle lay on my examination table in a state of stupor. No one was sure he would live or die. I didn't have any experience of handling snake bites. Yet, a GP cannot wash her hands off a patient. I knew I should try to the best of my capabilities and resources. I could see tiny marks of a bite on his right leg. One could not rely on the description of the distressed lad. His description of 'this long' could be just a foot-long snake. After a circuitous description of size and colour, I came to the conclusion that it was certainly not a cobra but could be a poisonous snake. I decided to give the man the precious antivenom shot from my fridge. He regained consciousness in a few moments.

I realised that such little awareness about reptile bites was not acceptable in a doctor.

Why did they not teach us about reptilian bites in detail? I started reading books on snakes and learnt about antivenom shots. I learnt the correct dosage of these shots and about the types of common snakes. I learnt how they looked and ways to identify them. It became easier once I could identify the snakes by the patient's description. I also discovered that snake antivenom serum was always in short supply in the country. Most people who died of snake bites either did not receive the antivenom or did not get enough of it. That started the trend of hoarding a few doses in my fridge at all times. It was these hoarded doses that saved so many lives over the years. Rats, monkeys, dogs and scorpion bites too were common. I never imagined that rats could be so adept and prolific at biting sleeping humans. Rats and monkey bites received the rabies shots.

Up until the 2000s, there was no talk of any litigation, so doctors could try and save lives without the fear of being sued. The patient was a person who needed help. One did not see him as a potential litigant; nor was a doctor treated like a potential criminal. When globalisation set in, people began to talk about suing doctors and taking them to court. My husband was on a medico-legal board as the surgical expert and knew the dangers of being sued.

Knowing that I had a penchant for valour in the clinic, he would drum some sanity into me, every single evening. He would tell me that only three things could save me from being sued—paperwork, paperwork and paperwork. Consequently, I started my journey of maintaining countless registers and spending more time getting signatures for every procedure I did. This was the beginning of times where a doctor spent more time managing paperwork than in seeing and treating patients. I gradually stopped trying to save lives.

Poisonings, accidents, snake bites, electrocutions and even breast abscesses were referred to Safdarjung Hospital. Anything that needed a call to my husband earlier was now referred to Safdarjung. Dreams of being a good doctor and maybe a heroic one flew out of the window. In spite of the mountains of paperwork, I like to believe that I saved many lives with this so-called foolhardiness in treating such cases. I called it responsibility.

The most horrific incident was when a man brought in a small child in his arms. His face was tear-stained; his clothes crumpled. As I gestured to him to lay the child on the table, he kept holding the limp body and crying inconsolably. He looked defeated and lost.

"What happened?" I asked.

"She was raped by the guard at the farm," he said amid sobs. "She was playing with the new ball I had bought for her." Just listening to him made my heart cry. The farm where the tragedy happened was a few yards away from the clinic. He had found her lying unconscious on the ground along with her muddy and blood-stained clothes. I cast a look at the child with her head hung loose over her father's shoulder. She looked about three years old. I did not meet the father's eyes for the grief and tears on his face were unbearable. I knew that the child was dead, yet I did the mandatory pupil test and auscultated her. I could see there were brutal tears and bruises on her body. Mechanically, I looked past his shoulder so as to not meet his eyes and said, "She is dead, I can't do anything." The father cried some more. I did not look at the child's face because I knew it would haunt me every night. He knew that it was a lost battle so he walked away, a sad, broken figure. I sat for a while, feeling sad. We owed it to our children to protect them and not fail them.

Why did we fail them?

This tragedy of the three-year-old was published in the newspapers the next morning, which made interesting headlines for the rest of the world. The genteel people of South Delhi clicked their sophisticated tongues and said, "How sad."

"The things that happen these days."

"Delhi is going to the dogs."

"Where are the police?"

"Did you hear about the three-year-old who was raped?"

All the right sounds were made and then they all went back to their lunches and parties. Did any tragedy ever permeate their perfumed exteriors? I wondered. Perhaps everything was forgotten in the gracefulness of their sanitised environs. I had lived in this same sophisticated environment until I was hurled over to the other side of the fence.

CHAPTER TEN

Was this a Miracle?

"There's no one thing that's true. It's all true".
Ernest Hemingway, *For Whom the Bell Tolls*

I WAS ALWAYS wary of unrealistic reverence because I knew how little it took for reverence to become revenge. Treating common colds and gastroenteritis was easy as one could always predict the time for recovery with great accuracy. To treat patients with unknown, undiagnosed and untreatable illnesses was very frightening. I knew that these rustic looking people were easily aroused. It took very little to make a mob out of them.

It was the summer of 1990. There was this case of an old man who was brought in by a regular patient whose diabetes I had managed to diagnose and control by proper medication and strict diet charts. There was no miracle involved here but the man insisted that I had performed one. So be it, I said to myself. As with most patients who got cured of chronic diseases like Diabetes, Tuberculosis, skin ailments and others, this one too became my brand ambassador. He would pop in every once in a while with one or two new patients in tow. I knew that he must be extolling unreal and exaggerated stuff about my medical prowess because the new patients he brought would have an embarrassingly worshipful air about them and sky-high expectations which worried me.

That day the so-called regular patient carried this old man in his arms like one would carry a sack of wheat.

"He is very sick but I know you can treat him," he said with a conviction that made me fearful. The man could not be made to sit on the stool as he was too weak. I gestured to the staff to help him lie down on the examination couch. As I approached him, he opened his eyes that were sunk deep in the orbits and his index finger pointed towards his mouth. I shone my torch inside his mouth. It was full of rotting ulcers. I could barely see anything else besides white sludge. He was absolutely emaciated. His skin hung loose on the bones. There was nothing more cadaveric I had ever seen except for real cadavers in the dissection room.

"He has not eaten a morsel in two years," said the man who had brought him. "He can only drink a cup of milk or water. The ulcers have been there for more than two years." The family were quietly seated all around on the benches. They looked up at me expectantly as if I would pull out a magic wand and wave it over their patient.

A youngish man carrying a large folder of medical records arose from the bench and handed those to me. I quickly went through them and saw that the patient had been to All India Institute of Medical Science in Delhi (AIIMS). This was the most respected tertiary care hospital in India. They had done a biopsy of the ulcers and the report clearly proclaimed, 'Malignant cells seen'.

So that was it. Where was my role after this?

"Take him back to AIIMS," I said almost in relief.

"No, no, Madam, you have to treat him. We know that only you can treat him," said the son. I could see that all the family had the same desperate plea in their eyes.

"We know that he will die. Please give him something. Just put your hand on his head," the wife implored in a meek, defeated voice and got up to touch my feet.

I shook my head and told them gently that nothing could be done for him. "Go back to the hospital and get radiotherapy," was all I could offer in terms of advice.

The old man's son replied, "We know nothing can cure him and that he will die." He paused for a moment to swallow the lump in his throat, and then continued, "Just give him something so that he has some hope in his last days, maybe a miracle will happen."

I shook my head in despair.

"Take him home then, there is no cure," I dissuaded them. If I hadn't read the diagnosis, maybe I would have relented. Knowing it was malignancy, how could I send him home with vitamin tablets?

"Please, please, give him just one tablet." The five pairs of eyes glued to my face wouldn't blink.

The son implored and bent down to touch my feet again. "Just give anything, please."

The wife stepped forward and said in a tone of finality, "We will take him home and not to the hospital," and she looked me straight in the eye. "Just make his life bearable so he can eat something till he lives."

I had no choice left. A decision had to be taken. I knew a

lot of patients with malignancies who went back home to live out the remainder of their lives.

I made a placebo-like concoction of tablets that included high doses of Vitamin B12, some steroids, a lot of Vitamin C and some mild antibiotics. I also added some Boroglycerine drops to be used hourly on the ulcers. This was the general treatment I gave for any oral ulcer. I decided to dispense this concoction for fifteen days. I could always refuse the treatment later, I thought to myself.

"Please give the medicines for at least two months," said the son. "We come from Rajasthan which is ten hours by road." Rajasthan was about 700 kilometres away. In those days of limited and inefficient transport options, it meant an easy ten hours commute one way and a few hundred rupees. I asked my staff to pack two months of the medicines for this old man and charged him a minimal amount as I was certain that nothing would come of it. I felt guilty charging for something which I knew wouldn't help so made up for my nagging guilt by a silent prayer for the old man. Two months later, one of the younger sons came again to get more medicines for yet another two months. I was hesitant but he was resolute so I caved in.

A day, sometime in June of 1990, it was a sultry afternoon and I was a bit exhausted from starting and managing endless IV lines for patients who had reported gastroenteritis. As I took a moment of respite, I saw this old man walking in. He was wearing a white kurta-pajama. He was gaunt and old but had a spring in his step and a smile on his face. As he entered my room, he bowed to say 'Namaste' to me and was about to touch my feet when I moved away and tucked them under my saree.

"Please sit down," I said hastily pointing towards the

patient's stool. As I fiddled with a file trying to look busy, two other men entered on his heels. One of them was carrying a big sack of something. "This is new wheat from our fresh harvest," he said proudly. "We got it for you; please accept madam."

The younger one became dewy-eyed as he said, "Thank you, doctor madam. You are God," he continued with reverence in his eyes, so naked that I shrank in my chair for I didn't know what it was about.

"You have performed a miracle," said the old man. "I don't think you recognise me," he continued, looking at my baffled expression.

Of course I didn't, I thought to myself. Why would I recognise him? I was sure I had never seen him before. I always remembered every patient that I saw.

The three men looked amused.

"He is the one who had cancer of the tongue," said the son quietly. "Your medicines have cured him. Look at him. He has no ulcers now… look… and he can eat." They were amused at my incredulous gaping.

Now that was impossible, I muttered in my mind. Somewhere there had to be a mistake.

I made the man sit on the stool and shone my torch in his mouth.

I was sure this was some rural belief. The mouth ulcers had to be there.

As I looked hard and turned the torch all around the mouth trying to find some evidence of ulceration or growth, I was surprised to see a clean mouth with not a whisper of an ulcer. I looked closely for something that looked like a small ulcer, redness or a malignant lesion.

"How? How could this happen?" I asked them bewildered. I knew I should have been asking this question to myself and not them. They were illiterate. How would they know?

"It's all your good treatment madam."

"It's not possible, take him to AIIMS; maybe it has regressed temporarily."

Then the son took out a file.

"We took him to All India Institute where they had tested him earlier."

As I held the report of the biopsy that read 'No malignant cells seen', I was confused. Obviously the earlier report was wrong. There had to be some scientific explanation. I was happy that this man, who would have died of starvation, was well now. After all, I was here to make people well. I knew Father would be proud of me.

As the word of 'the miracle' got around I started getting patients who required real miracles. This opened another plethora of ailments—ailments that no doctor is equipped to deal with. It was difficult to contain these cases. Luckily, most of these cases were of neglected infections. I could deal with these, without drawing on my non-existent magical powers. Some that did have a proven disease but got cured remain a mystery for they defied all scientific logic and medical books.

One of these was the case of another old man.

He was brought to me on a stretcher. He had had a road accident a few weeks back and his back was broken. They carried his X-rays that had been done in a well-known spinal centre. The X-rays showed fracture of the spine at the L 5 level along with a few ribs that were fractured, too. I told the relatives to take him to the All India Institute. That was the only place in the country that could treat such complex fractures.

“No, we have come to you to get treated,” said the son.

“This is stupidity,” I retaliated sharply.

“If you don’t treat him, we will take him home. Let God decide his fate,” said the son with finality in a no-nonsense tone. I knew that they would do exactly that because no one wanted to go to big hospitals.

I was aware that the spinal injuries could come around and start improving in a few weeks.

When the family refused to leave the clinic till I gave the old man my medicines, I had no choice. I put this man on a lot of B complex, some anti-inflammatory drugs and a good diet. I advised them to lay him flat on a semi-hard bed.

The son agreed to let me know the prognosis once a month.

A month later, the son walked in. I searched his face nervously to deduce the prognosis.

He smiled and said, “Well, my father can sit up a bit and he can also move his legs slightly.” I knew that it was the natural healing of the nerves taking place. “We have come to take more of the same medicines for another month.”

I realised once again the tremendous power of placebos. Never again would I scoff at them. It’s very unfashionable to use terms like faith and placebos in high-end medical care, yet I came to swear by these terms. It’s gratifying to know that hundreds of patients have gone back to living a healthy life when all I did was offer them a nice chat and some placebos nicely packed, with all good intentions and in all seriousness.

One month later when the son came again, his smile was wider and I could detect a sense of wonderment on his face.

“My father can sit up and eat now, thank you madam.” His

eyes were moist with gratitude. I repeated the same medicine as I knew it must have been a time-bound improvement of the nerves.

CHAPTER ELEVEN

The Reluctant Gynaecologist

"You have to take risks. We will only understand the miracle of life fully when we allow the unexpected to happen".

Paulo Coelho

WHEN SELECTING RESIDENCIES, most of my friends opted for gynaecology as everyone was aware that gynaecology was the most remunerative field. Female doctors by their gender were expected to be gynaecologists and it was easy to set-up an obstetrics practice.

I had developed such a dislike for this field that I never even considered it as an option. I was used to having a choice—always. As we chatted in the long corridors of the hospital, I patted myself for making smart choices for I was sure that I was never going to work in this field. Gynaecology was not for me. Paediatrics was elite and my joy, so I selected a Paediatric residency in Kalawati Saran Children's Hospital; not for me the pedestrian gynaecology practice.

The complacency of youth is surely misplaced.

Once in the clinic it was presumed by my patients that I was a gynaecologist. I resisted initially and told them I wasn't one. As the years passed, the stream of women patients kept becoming longer and the number of children became fewer by comparison. Hence, the mantle of gynaecology wrapped itself suffocatingly around me. I had no choice. Gradually, as I tread deeper into this specialty, reading and asking colleagues, I learnt the intricacies of this field. Mostly I learnt from my patients. I recorded the treatment and its results and learnt on the way. I had not completed a residency in gynaecology so whenever I examined a case, I felt like an imposter.

I had been accepted in Kapashera and all the neighbouring villages as a successful infertility specialist. Then women started to fill my clinic with diseases specific to women. I did not mind treating abdominal pains, cramps and urinary infections. Delayed periods, irregular periods and late or early menarche crept insidiously into my practice. It was inevitable that unwanted pregnancies too were not far behind but I did not have the expertise to deal with them. I avoided them for a year or two. The internal examinations became a nuisance. How could they know the intense dislike I had for internal examinations? When they insisted, I found excuses to avoid examining them. "You come next week, I will definitely examine you nicely; I am really in a hurry today."

"You take this medicine and I will examine you after that."

"It may cause pain if I examine you today, let me do it on the next visit." These were some of the excuses I raked up. However, there were situations when I ran out of excuses and could not avoid internal examinations. There were fibroids, infections and intrauterine contraceptive devices that had to be checked. All of them jarred my senses. I resisted, refused and referred most of those patients to other doctors in Gurgaon. Soon I was sending back most patients untreated.

Suddenly, the irony dawned on me that I was here to treat patients and not send them back because of my fanciful longings and my own biases. I was handling primary health care, and sending the patients back was counterproductive to my cause.

I steeled myself and enrolled in a six-month certificate course for Gynaecology procedures. Armed with the certificate, I confidently set out to perform all Gynaecology procedures. At least, now I did not feel like an imposter. The difficult cases, of course, were referred to a nursing home. After a while, I began to treat infertility, pap smears, multiload insertions, antenatal care and, of course, early pregnancies. Amidst globalisation unwanted pregnancies rose like a deluge, engulfing my practice. As the wave of modernisation caught the young population, they adopted western lifestyles. Of course, they were not armed to deal with the after effects of a late night date, which is true the world over.

The most vulnerable and least protected population falls victim to any changes in society and is always the worst hit.

There would be at least five or six young, unmarried girls, waiting every single day in the waiting room for medical termination of unwanted pregnancy. I was prepared for this procedure as I had trained in what is called Menstrual Regulation at the Indo-British NGO, Marie Stopes International. I learnt about contraception, abortions and planned parenthood. My six-month training in their centre armed me with enough practical experience to deal with most of my Gynaecology patients. In addition to this training, the large number of patients, too, provided me with a learning platform.

The inherent resistance to practising Gynaecology still

remains, but I do understand that in a general practice, one cannot avoid it. Even after decades of practising gynaecology, I have misgivings each time I see a patient with a gynaecology-related problem.

One thing that is close to my heart is family planning. I feel very strongly about the ideal family with two kids, but I realised that the number of children a woman ought to have was rarely the couple's decision. The mother-in-law, the man's sisters, the neighbours and the relatives from other villages, all had opinions about sterilisation. To convince one person was easy but to convince forty people was an ordeal. I never tired of the counselling sessions even if it meant multiple sessions for each of them. One happy patient meant a few more from the same village, then many more.

The government offered incentives and paid the Anganwadi workers (village social health workers) a small amount for every patient brought in for a tubectomy. In spite of these efforts by the government, all the five-year plans for population control failed miserably for the simple reason that people needed to take a day off to go to the hospital. The labour drain from villages was at an all-time high so availability of labour was high. Even if a man took one day's leave, he was laid-off.

When the logistics of going to Marie Stopes didn't work for a couple, the husbands would convince their wives to continue with the pregnancy saying that the child was God's gift. It was no wonder that God was generous with his gifts of endless babies in India. Too many babies caused so much havoc and cast the curse of poverty over millions of people. I knew that if the government had legalised a few days of paid leave for family planning needs, the population numbers would tell a different story.

I hadn't cultivated anyone in the administrative circles but I wish I had. Perhaps I should have attended those conferences and conventions in air-conditioned halls. Maybe, I wouldn't have had a say in any policies since I didn't have too many degrees on my visiting card. But if invited, I could have exchanged some meaningful notes with people who sat around big tables, sipping mineral water and enjoying the sandwiches and samosas at the tea service. These policymakers and doctors in the conference rooms were so far removed from reality, that they didn't have a clue about real poverty, drudgery and slavery that changed the sickness patterns and medical needs of the people. Making lofty policies based on graphs far removed from real life was completely ineffectual. Maybe I should have tried harder to get into these hallowed circles.

A solution had to be found where the husband did not need to take leave for his wife's tubectomy. I got in touch with some of the Anganwadi workers who were local village women and shared a great camaraderie with the villagers. I paid the Anganwadi worker some sweat money so she could take the patient to the hospital, fill in the paperwork, stay with her throughout the procedure and get her tea if she needed. She could hire an auto rickshaw and get her home after the operation, and also stay with her till her husband returned from work. Men started to come with their wives and inquire about the details of the whole procedure, and were happy to pay an extra amount to the social worker. It was an insubstantial amount but the benefits were incalculable. That way, the husband did not need to take a day off work. After the operation, the social worker visited the patient daily for five days to check the stitches and to make sure all was okay. The uneventful post-op period was extremely important for the acceptance of this procedure. I knew that just one post-op complication could jeopardise the success of the tubectomy procedure. In no time, I had an army of enthusiastic social workers who worked for a small pittance, which added up to a substantial amount because they received some amount from the government agencies too. Everyone was happy with the arrangement.

There were a few women who were so driven that they went without telling the husband. Doing so was perfectly legal as anyone with more than two children did not need the husband to sign on the dotted line.

I wish the government had realised that thousands of babies were born because missing a day at work was unacceptable to most daily wagers.

The shining hope for family planning came in the form of liberalisation. With liberalisation came hundreds of garment-export units. They needed thousands of hands to make and finish the garments—snipping errant threads and sewing buttons needed female acumen. As more and more women joined the workforce, they looked better and healthier. The garment business boomed, and soon, almost every household had women working in the factories. I witnessed the effects on these women, from being unemployed to being employed.

They could afford medical care and send their children to school. It had an effect on the level of their children's education and health parameters. When the women went to work, there were improvements in the diet of the family and consequently, reduction in sickness episodes. Their employment had an impact on the number of children they had. Having more than two children was not acceptable to the couples anymore because a pregnancy would disrupt the woman's job and the second income would be lost. It just became so natural for a couple to go in for contraceptive devices. People and the press were so busy harping about the failed population control plans that no one celebrated this small victory of small families. Women's employment was another factor that was overlooked. Had government policymakers recognised this fact and offered more jobs to women, our population would have shown more promising results in health and fertility indices.

By 2010, most families consisted of two children as opposed to four or five, and a sizeable number of families had two-income streams.

The same figures reflected in abortions, too. In the late nineties, when the garment export factories mushroomed, armies of women were employed. One could see these women making their way to the factory sheds every morning. They could be seen in swarms running for the buses, taking urgent, hurried steps in their sarees. They had to reach on time. If they were even a minute late, they would lose half a day's salary.

They were women, so they had women's problems, and they obviously got pregnant at some point. A few of them confided that the managers had a big say in who would be laid off and who would be promoted. Some of these women tried the easy channels to climb up the ladder. It was natural that unwanted pregnancies multiplied. The hapless woman would come alone or with a female friend, from work, for an abortion. They got an hour for lunch, so I would do the MR procedure in less than five to ten minutes. After resting for thirty minutes, they could go back to work just in time when the lunch break ended.

It was rarely that they came in with the husband. I knew

what was happening. I did not judge, comment or pronounce any verdict, but I could guess the genesis of these pregnancies. Some women would tell me in confidence that the manager had misbehaved with them.

"Please don't tell my husband," was the only request because they knew that the husband would put a stop to their work and independence.

I found myself deeply involved in gynaecology and obstetrics; it was a miracle that I was spared the agony of birthing because it was more than I could deal with. I called the patients for ANC (Antenatal check-up) for nine months and then referred them to a good obstetrician for the delivery. In spite of being careful not to get involved in birthing, a few women managed to give birth in my waiting room, much to my chagrin.

It was early morning when Somwati, a new patient I had never set eyes on, came to the clinic, just as a member of my staff opened the shutters. Her husband in tow, she was full-term pregnant. I had just reached the clinic. Roopa came in to tell me that Somwati was complaining of severe abdominal pain. Alarm bells rang in my ears.

"Refer her to Safdarjung," I instructed curtly without getting up from my chair. She could go to some hospital. My clinic was definitely not a birthing centre.

"But…but…she…."

"Just go and let her out." I quickly cut her short. And that was the end of the matter or so I thought. As I got up a few minutes later to take stock of the situation, I was aghast and panic-stricken to see the fully pregnant patient lying on one of the benches in my waiting room, with her husband sitting beside her rubbing her tummy. She was wailing and screaming in pain.

"You need to take her to the hospital."

"We can't go to the hospital," said the husband.

"How many children do you have?" I asked hopefully. If it was the first child, she still had some time to deliver and I could convince them to go to Safdarjung Hospital. I prayed hard that it was her first child.

"Four," came the prompt reply.

Oh my, I said to myself. Before I could gather my thoughts, the feisty cry of a newborn filled my waiting room. Flustered, panic-stricken and incredulous, I quickly fetched my forceps and a new blade to clinch and cut the cord. Luckily, there were no other patients to witness my lack of expertise. The patient, the baby and the waiting room were cleaned and mopped up thoroughly. Safe in my arms, the baby was smiling as if it had achieved some great feat. A great feat no doubt for it had gained an unwelcome entry in my clinic.

Many people commented that the baby being born in my waiting room was a sign that I should start a birthing centre, but I was adamant. "Why don't you start admitting pregnant patients; you can make tons of money just birthing babies?" said a few well-meaning friends. I would look at them and smile. "I don't want to earn tons of money," I would say, bored of their logic. I really meant it for I had no use of any extra money doing Gynae or Obstetrics.

Over the years, I had just one more unintended and unexpected delivery in my waiting room, which was comical in its timing too. The patient, Ramadi, had been coming to the clinic for ANC for a few months and on this day, she decided to visit me for a final check-up. As she alighted from the hand-pulled rickshaw, she got a sudden uterine contraction and squealed in pain. My staff peeped out as her husband helped her to walk into the clinic. Before she could enter the clinic, the baby found its way into the hands of the father. I could only smile as I saw him hold the baby with one hand, still attached to the cord, and steady his wife with the other. Again, out came my forceps and surgical blade. These two incidents were aberrations. Birthing was completely unthinkable for me.

Of course, I had the X-ray machine, which I used for Hysterosalpingograms (HSG).

As I gained more confidence, I started doing Hysterosalpingograms regularly for infertility. I was on familiar ground with this one investigation that was key to the treatment of infertility. I made many modifications along the way in gynaecology practice; I failed in some and won others. For the HSGs, I experimented with a finer IUI cannula to insert the dye into the uterus. The use of this fine cannula made the procedure a cakewalk for me and almost painless for the patient. It was sheer luck that my patients started to conceive faster after I did their Hysterosalpingogram. Gradually, as the stone crushers in Rajokri closed down, safety standards became better and tuberculosis and fractures were fewer, but I found my X-ray machine stayed busy with just hysterosalpingograms.

There are many times in a medical practice when it seems very easy to be a little bit dishonest. At these times, dishonesty seems natural and the simplest way out rather than face an irate patient. It looks tempting because the patient would never know what procedure had been done. In my experience, one has to be honest with oneself and the patient for long-term benefits. There were many cases where the temptation to lie just a little bit came my way. Since I wasn't a natural at gynaecology, I had many moments of doubt and uncertainty.

If a HSG did not come out well, I had a choice like any other doctor. I could tell the patient that I had seen both the uterine tubes clearly and send her away happily or I could admit that she would need to come back for a repeat HSG.

I had to be honest to Father.

There was no way I was going to let him down. On the many occasions when I could not diagnose the symptoms or the cause of excessive bleeding, I knew that I needed to consult a colleague. I would come home and read journals, and ask colleagues till I found the right answer.

When there is no risk of getting caught, that is the crucial time that one has to be honest. When one knows that the risk of getting caught is high, there is no honesty at all. That's how characters get built.

A patient, Gopal, a short Nepalese with chinky eyes that were filled with warmth, came from Nepal just to be treated for infertility. "You are famous in our village in Nepal," he said simply. "There are so many couples who have conceived with your help," he said. That I made a permanent dent in people's lives sustained me, even if it meant making peace with a Gynaecology practice.

A couple who had been married for more than twenty years comes to mind. They had no children so his wife was the target of ridicule, abuse and mocking in the village. In a country where a man's manhood is measured by the number of children he sires, the husband had had enough of being heckled with taunts and jeers. After being treated for infertility for a few months the lady missed a period. When I put the urine on the test strip, it showed two lines indicating a pregnancy. The man was overwhelmed; he could not contain his joy and went out for a few minutes as he wept unabashedly in the waiting room. Uncontrollable tears, the grateful look and the disbelief on their faces was more than I deserved. Of course, I was just a medium for these miraculous acts.

Only God can take credit for such rewards! Such miracles started to take place quite frequently and I received the glory and adulation with great humility. I knew that these joys would remain long after I was gone.

Who can ever be sure of what the future holds for us? There came a point after 2010 when most children seemed to be healthy except for erratic colds and coughs. My persistent advice of using boiled water, eating fresh food and completing all vaccination schedules got results that were a GP's dream. As the children whittled out of my practice, the clinic saw increasing footfalls of women patients. It was obvious that I was completely entrenched in a gynaecology practice.

How did this happen?

How did I let it happen?

I had to do some good and I had to change lives. Wasn't that what had brought me here? I adopted Gynaecology or maybe it was the other way around. Gynaecology adopted me and became the mainstay of my practice. As I saw the rows of patients waiting in the outside room with Gynaecological ailments, my heart would sink. It still sinks. I was doing just that one thing that I never wanted to do—Gynaecology!

My son had become conversant with modes of doing business after a few years in corporate finance. He would cajole me into selling franchises for my clinic.

"Make it scalable, Mom," he would persist. "You are popular, sell the name." But I never had the desire to scale it up. To go back to the privileged side was possible had I made an effort earlier, but quite insidiously there had crept in a discomfort with wealth. It was not a new feeling. Even as a student, there were days when I would leave my car at home and take a bus to college with other classmates because I wanted to be like everyone else. When in Kapashera, I saw so much poverty and need that the privileged life which was mine, stuck out like a sore spot. It no longer enticed or excited me.

CHAPTER TWELVE

All about Bad Milk

A STRANGE POWER game was being played in most households.

Close observations revealed unexpected facets of joint families.

The male baby was the star attraction. He belonged to the whole family. The mother of this baby was an outsider and had no investment in the baby. The mother-in-law or sister-in-law wanted total power over this male child; the battle was all about the son or the grandson while the mother of the child became a worker bee, completely irrelevant.

"Your milk is not good for the baby."

"The milk is not enough, the baby keeps crying."

"The baby falls sick whenever you hold him."

"You should just do the cooking and cleaning, I will hold the baby."

With the constant drumming and ridiculing, the mother started to believe that her milk was not good enough for her son. She was not allowed to breastfeed or even hold the baby. She would be assigned unending household work while the baby gurgled and cooed in the mother-in-law's lap and was bottle-fed while the mother became irrelevant in everyone's lives. The young mothers often broke into inexplicable tears. No one knew why they cried, and they themselves did not know why they were so unhappy.

It was a very delicate nuance, difficult to perceive by the husbands and fathers. After I recognised the dynamics of power, I figured out the cause of the unshed tears as these new mothers came with non-specific symptoms. Their faces wore a perpetual sad look and they did not realise what was happening to them. It was too subtle. The mothers blamed themselves for their unhappiness, their grievances, their headaches, their backaches and everything else. They felt they were not good enough for the family and for their baby. The mothers-in-law blamed them, the neighbours blamed them and the husbands wrung their hands in despair. The poor husband was completely unaware of the fight for power going on right under his nose, while it wreaked permanent havoc on the young mother's psyche. It was easy to detect a pattern in this whole process.

This behaviour occurred only when a male child was involved.

I spent hours of consultation and counselling to convince the husband and give hope and strength to the distraught woman. Most of the time, my counselling had no effect and did not change their deep-rooted beliefs. I continued relentlessly and encouraged them to breastfeed. Weighing the baby every time they came in, I showed the mothers-in-law that the baby was gaining good weight when breastfed. It was the mother-in-law who was, invariably, the supreme force in the family, and I learnt gradually that if I had to get anywhere with any patient, I had to be in her good books. If a patient had to visit me again to complete a course of UTI or PID, it was my job to impress upon the mother-in-law and convince her that in the long run, this thing may give trouble. Conviction, cajoling, compliments and reasoning, all came in useful.

The young mothers of that time are now mothers-in-law, and have an unquestionable faith in me. When their daughters-in-law get pregnant, they visit me with hope and trust.

"She is all yours to manage. You take care of her for nine months."

Coming back to the game of power in the house, breastfeeding advice worked for some and they relented. The weight-taking became so popular that many mothers came in just to weigh their child. I knew it was less about the baby and more of a confidence boost for themselves.

Many mothers suffered from postpartum depression, which was unheard of in those times. In fact, even today, families look disdainfully and incredulously if I mention postpartum depression. No one believes it is an entity. The diagnosis and treatment has to be done covertly and without fee as no money can be expected from the husband anyway for something like postpartum depression. I know how devastating it can be as I, too, suffered from depression soon after the birth of my daughter. I felt worthless, ugly and incompetent, even though I ran a busy practice. I never had the confidence to mention it to my husband. I looked sick and gaunt because I lost more than twenty pounds that year. And no one noticed. It was the busy clinic that saved me from the darkness and gloom. Once again, I thanked Father for his gift of the clinic.

CHAPTER THIRTEEN

Histories and Stories

HISTORY TAKING IS the backbone of any medical practice, especially in a rural set-up where just finding out the date of the last menstrual period is like calculating the speed of light.

An old professor of Medicine used to say this in all his lectures. History taking and palpitation, he would say, were the two most important things in diagnosis. He repeated this in every class. We never took him seriously and discarded his words as 'old fogey' ideas.

Later in my clinic, I realised that asking for the colour of a baby's stool saved many a day. The colour helped me to differentiate between a bacterial infection that needed antibiotics and a viral infection that needed nothing besides extra water. Years and years of asking for the colour of the stool, as if my life depended on it, trained my patients too.

"What is the colour?"

"How many times?"

"Since when?"

They would come prepared to answer my questions.

During the decades in the clinic, I have seen many patients who came back to me after consulting super-specialists. I find that these specialists have missed the simplest diagnosis by ignoring the history-taking step. I have seen patients being admitted to big private hospitals for fever. When they don't get cured, I see that they haven't even been tested for typhoid. Once correctly diagnosed they would recover in five-six days at a fraction of the cost. A simple chest X-ray, which many doctors missed doing, could diagnose pneumonia, which was very common. Proper treatment of fifteen days would get them up and about. This was all without any hospitalisation.

Some histories took the cake. Simple questions like, "How many children do you have?"

"Two."

The neighbour who had come with this one looked at her and whispered, "You have four, don't you?"

I heard the whisper, "four", and looked at both of them perplexed. Seeing that there was a long queue of patients getting restless in the waiting room, I knew I had to hurry up or those patients would leave.

"If you count the ones in the village," she tapered off, still undecided.

"How many have you produced?" I asked sharply.

She looked around and then a bit sheepishly she said, "Ok, so I think then it should be six." She was still counting on her fingers.

"Two are with me, two are in the village with my mother," she stopped to think and then, "two girls are married."

"Why didn't you tell me earlier?" I asked looking annoyed.

"The girls are in their own homes, so why should I count

them?" she pouted. "We don't count married girls."

I was surprised at the number of women who had a 'history'—a history of teen pregnancies, history of multiple abortions and history of elopements. The surprise was because these girls were from a rural background and did not have access to any modern clothes or accessories to entice the boys.

A patient, Meenu, who was pretty and newly-married, wore shiny, new bangles, a silver lace-lined long shirt, an embroidered salwar and very bright lipstick, which was normal for a newlywed. Her brand new husband sat outside in the waiting room. She had come to visit me because she was pregnant.

"How many months have you been married?" I quizzed casually.

"Three months," she replied coyly.

On examination of her abdomen, I felt that the fetal lump was about twenty weeks. Maybe I was mistaken but I could swear that I felt the fetal movements.

Maybe she had forgotten her dates.

Maybe what I suspected was not true. "Okay, so let's get an ultrasound done." I hoped that I was wrong and the pregnancy would be not more than twelve weeks.

The ultrasound centre sent their van to collect Meenu. An hour later she came back with her ultrasound in her hand.

"I think there has been some mistake," I said as I saw her report. The report showed a pregnancy of five months. Maybe they had mixed her film with someone else's.

"I'll just call the doctor in the lab."

"Why, what happened?"

"Are you sure you got married three months ago?" I asked her.

"Yes, I am sure," she said firmly with a defiant look in her eyes. Then she walked over to my table and whispered in a very low voice, "Can I tell you something?"

"Of course," I said, knowing what to expect.

She whispered in my ear, "You know, I had a boyfriend in the village but I was not allowed to marry him," she said in a conspiratorial tone, pausing for a moment to gauge my reaction, expecting me to look suitably shocked.

I do wish sometimes that I had lesser insight.

"Oh, that explains the eight-week gap." I looked as nonchalant as Meenu about this piece of information. Anyway, a reaction from me would solve no purpose. "Oh, okay, let me see how we manage it."

"Please don't tell my husband," she pleaded. "He will leave me if he gets to know."

The dilemma of whether to tell or not to tell bothered me yet once again. I reasoned the same way as before. The girl who sat in front of me was my patient and I had to prioritise her interests.

"I will not offer the truth to your husband," I told her, "but if he asks me directly, I will not lie to him either," I said conclusively. That was a good stand, I thought.

"Thank you, doctor," she looked relieved. "I will make sure he waits in the waiting room every time I visit you." Meenu was smiling in relief and I felt like a co-conspirator to her village frolic.

Even in the present, modern times, I feel the conundrum of 'to tell or not to tell' has no correct answer. It can be debated in many ways. A husband's right to know and many other paternity issues would crop up if someone were to rip the issue apart just for discussion's sake. I had many cases before Meenu and after Meenu. Cases where the gestation period did not match the last menstrual period. I chose to keep quiet and believed that it was the patient's right to tell or not to tell. Who was I to break up a marriage? After all, she was an adult. According to my Hippocratic Oath I was being loyal to my patient and the woman has the right over her body.

One of my favourite and regular patients is an autorickshaw *wala* (as they are called). They drive the ubiquitous three-wheeler autos that teem the streets of Delhi. Mohanlal was one of the thousands of insignificant autorickshaw drivers. He was thin and gaunt, his cheeks were sunken and his eyes were always downcast in humility. He always entered the clinic with an apologetic and hesitant smile as if he was sorry to disturb me. If he saw that I was busy, he and his family would wait in the autorickshaw. His wife Sheela, and two daughters aged fifteen and seventeen, were also regulars at my clinic with the usual problems of dysmenorrhea, colds and coughs. Somehow, they always managed to pool their ailments and come together, so that one ride to the clinic would suffice for the whole family. That would save Mohanlal the loss of a working day. Sheela was a school teacher and our rickshaw driver was a school dropout. With a wide educational difference in the couple, I found them to be an interesting case study. Whenever they came to my clinic, I looked at their faces to study the couple dynamics. That is the reason why this couple has found their way to these pages. That particular day, the daughters were not in the autorickshaw. I beckoned them to sit opposite my table so they could face me.

Sheela was unusually quiet on this particular day; her face

devoid of her customary smile she sat with her head bowed low. I wondered why and waited patiently for the events to unfurl.

"Yes?" I said to start a conversation.

"You know how difficult life is," said Mohanlal, looking past at the wall behind me.

I was baffled by Mohanlal's demeanour.

He moved nearer to my table. He bent forward so my staff could not hear anything. "Please help me."

"Oh, so she is pregnant," I said in obvious enlightenment.

"Yes, she is pregnant," he was barely audible.

"That's ok, there's no need to be so embarrassed," I said to allay his apprehensions.

"No, no, it's not mine," he blurted out in agony. "She went to her village and met her old friend over there."

I was incredulous at the fact that the simple-looking, middle-aged school teacher could fall prey to the charms of a village Romeo and this naive auto driver carried no angst at his wife's adulterous behaviour. To say that I was taken aback would be a euphemism. This was the most sedate and devoted couple I had come across in years. I cast a look at Sheela as she sat with her head bent low, clearly sorry and mortified to the core, wishing she could disappear into the floor, and then at Mohanlal who sat confused trying to justify his wife's waywardness. I looked at him in disbelief as I waited for him to show some human frailty. Maybe he would confess his anger and disappointment at this betrayal. I wanted him to fall to a human level. This was adultery and betrayal. How was he so calm and accepting? But there were no hidden or covert signals that conveyed anger, agitation or angst.

At that moment, I knew I had seen the best example of

forgiveness ever. This was a fine human being, an illiterate auto driver. All my life I thought that education refined humans. Did it? I wasn't sure now.

"Just make her okay again," he said softly, completely at terms with himself and the situation. "She is my wife," he continued in a passive voice that meant let bygones be bygones, let me not lose my ideal life.

"Everyone can make mistakes," he said. Not a hint of patronising or of martyrdom. Never once did he look at her accusingly. I looked at him in admiration—admiration for his forbearance, self-control and submission to reality. I could never envisage such acceptance of a spouse's betrayal even in the so-called liberal circles.

I quickly performed the procedure and they went on their way in his autorickshaw. This was many years ago.

I learnt my lesson in forgiveness and that it's a virtue that builds lifelong bonds.

CHAPTER FOURTEEN

The Girl's Period or a Curse

HER PERIOD WAS so important for everyone. I realised this as I heard stories from my female patients and their menfolk. Mother gave no importance to periods and I grew up unaware of its importance in society—playing, running, racing, because it was just like getting a cold. It came and went away. It was in Kapashera that I realised how important an event it was. Daily lives, school attendance, marriages, festivals, religious functions, social interactions and everything else was governed by a girl's menstrual cycle.

Naumi or the ninth day of the rising moon which involved nine days of fasting was a popular festival when people would end their fast by a ceremony which included inviting young girls (*kanya*), who had not yet started menstruating, for a feast. They would be worshipped by the women of the family and given gifts of money and clothes. This tradition is practised over the country by all—literate and illiterate! Even in modern India, it's practised widely. A girl was looked at in a different light if she had started her periods. Before menarche she was pure and could be worshipped but the moment she started her periods she became impure. The mores and restrictions that were imposed on her were callous and unimaginable. I learnt about these practices from my staff girls, who were village girls and were subjected to these rules themselves. They had seen their mothers following these rules and there was no question of them not following their mothers.

"I can't enter the kitchen when I have my period," said Seema, one of my staff. "My food is different from my brother's; I get a separate plate when I have my period." It was most natural for them. The girls were made to sleep on the floor in the spare storeroom and they never thought of complaining. They couldn't put their fingers in the pickle jar as the pickle would get spoiled. They couldn't wash their hair during those days as it was a bad omen for the brothers. They couldn't go out of the house to meet friends. They couldn't serve food to the father or the brothers for their lives could be endangered, especially if her gaze fell on them during her period. They couldn't visit a temple because God would get angry and curse the entire family. Attending a religious ceremony during periods was sacrilege and would bring disaster to the whole village. In short, they were denigrated to the lowest level while they bore the cross of the period. I cringed at the thought that a young girl's periods were family and community knowledge. With so many rules and restrictions, the girls lost their verve to sing, scamper and pirouette.

Where was the joy of girlhood?

Where were the giggles and the laughter?

They became sedate, solemn and introverted, a desired trait in girls. They became women at thirteen!

One of my staff girls was from the hilly regions. A feisty girl! Her feistiness had not been tampered with, in spite of the restrictions that were laid by her new mother-in-law. I loved her for it. One day I noticed that she looked a bit low. "Tara, what happened?" I knew she was young and newly-married. She started to sob in her dupatta.

"It's okay, come here and tell me what happened."

"My mother-in-law doesn't let me sleep on the bed."

"Why not?" I asked casually.

"Whenever I have my periods, I have to sleep on the floor," she said in a loud protest. "My father gave me that bed," a pause was followed by more snivelling. "Why can't I sleep on that bed?" She looked at me expectantly, waiting for a reaction.

"I can't cook for my husband, I can't talk to him; I can't go out with him and I can't even bathe during those days." I had never seen this calm girl so flustered before. "My mother-in-law called me today to make sure that I was not cooking for my husband because she says he will fall sick."

I asked her to bring her husband over so I could convince him about the pain he was inflicting on the girl. As it turned out, the husband was an amenable young man, as intimidated by his mother as his young wife. It didn't take much for him to see the inhumane side of the rules thrust upon his new bride.

"These are modern times so let the mother-in-law learn new rules," I added as a parting rejoinder. This brought a smile on their strained faces.

How much ignorance and falsity is there in these practices! Maybe it was a power game to keep the patriarchs unthreatened and unchallenged.

The unnatural interest in the periods of women manifested

itself in sexual abuse of young girls. Since everyone made a girl's menstrual cycle their business, it wasn't surprising that a woman was considered public property. A logical mind can deduce the origin of the *sindoor* and the red bangles that a married woman has to wear. If the woman is married, she is someone else's property and no male can cast his gaze upon her. The red sindoor in the hair alerts all males from a mile away. An unmarried girl is fodder for all.

As I stood with Baburam one afternoon inspecting the new room which was getting added to the clinic, he murmured almost inaudibly, "You should do a small puja, Madam." I turned to look at him. I knew he was thinking of Father who always lit a *diya* for new beginnings. My heart yearned for my father.

"I don't have any puja things," I said, half hoping he would forget about it. "Just get a candle and light it," he continued matter-of-factly. "Give some sweets to a young girl who hasn't had her periods." I was aghast and furious that a girl's right to sweets was according to her periods. I looked away without a word.

"There is one, look," he said excitedly, pointing to a young girl of five who was playing hopscotch with a friend in the house opposite the clinic. "She is young and couldn't have had her periods." Baburam was illiterate, yet he was conversant with the biology of the female. It made me seethe in disgust at the public scrutiny of a girl's most private life.

Taking the menstrual history from veiled village women was a test of one's patience. Just to find out about the date of the last menstrual period was like running around in circles. To make matters worse, she was always accompanied by her brother-in-law, her father-in-law, father-in-law's brothers, her sister, her sister's husband and his brother, the neighbour, the neighbour's brother and at the bottom of the hierarchy would be her timid husband. When asked how regular her period was, they would all answer at once. I never knew who to look at to get my answer. The half a dozen people who stood surrounding her would be agitating silently, like a class of eager boys waiting to raise their hand and be the first to provide the answer. The men's vast knowledge about her menstruation cycle both amused and angered me. All this while the lady would sit completely veiled, her head lost somewhere in her dupatta.

So there was this patient, a young bride, who came to me one winter morning. "Can you see if she is pregnant?" rasped the oldish woman who accompanied her. She was authoritative in her demeanour. As I took stock, I saw that there was a conglomeration of assorted men, some in crumpled kurtas and others in fresh ones, just behind her, peeping curiously and trying to hear my words. I gestured for them to leave the room and wait outside.

"When was your last period?" There was complete silence. The only movement was of the rustle of the shiny saree that swathed her head which was moving in a half-nodding, half-shaking movement.

"Why is she not answering?"

"She is shy," the mother-in-law stated as a fact.

"Sixteenth of last month," one of the men answered from outside. He was clearly eavesdropping.

"No, no, it was on the twentieth," another voice, louder, ruled over the first one.

"You all don't know, it was on the first," another authoritative voice, even louder, rang across the consultation room. I looked towards this voice appalled out of my composure. I wondered how the neighbours, in-laws, brothers and everyone else got so involved with a woman's menstrual history while she was not considered mature enough to mention her own dates.

"Do you remember the dates?" I asked the new bride gently.

"When I went to the village." The barely audible answer didn't help either. It made me more confused than ever. Never mind, I said to myself, let's find out when she went to the village.

"When did you go to the village?"

"Diwali."

Diwali was easy to locate on the calendar.

My staff girls scurried to find a calendar to look up the date for Diwali in the year. Armed with the Diwali date, I confronted her, "Diwali was three months ago."

"So you haven't had your period for three months?" I asked tightly as I was losing my patience.

"No, I got it once again when I came back from the village." I was ready to swear in frustration but took a deep breath to calm my nerves as we were back to where we started.

"When did you get back from the village?" I continued.

"I don't remember," she said looking exhausted at the volley of questions and quickly lost interest in me. As I fretted and fumed, she started to examine the bright, chipped orange nail polish on her nails.

Looking in exasperation at my staff girls, I saw one of them make her way out to tackle the all-knowing five men, who had accompanied the new bride. They would know the right answer, of course. In about five minutes, my assistant got the precious dates from them and came back with a gloating look on her face.

"She got it fifteen days after Diwali," she announced victoriously.

I must've spent more than half my career in extracting the correct menstrual history. Grilling the patient relentlessly always led to surprising results.

CHAPTER FIFTEEN

Travelling along NH 8

TODAY NH 8 is a dream run. One can zip down the eight-lane highway. No airport runway could be better. I write about it because NH8 is a very important part of my life. I must've spent half my waking time on this highway. I have watched endless sunsets and been bewitched by the languorous moon on this stretch while driving to and fro from the evening clinic. Driving through a fine drizzle that covered my windshield in a soft embrace, passionate thunderstorms that raked up dormant stories and romances, roaring winds and distracting shadows cast by a full moon that stirred the heart, made my drives a bit less mundane. The moon that followed me from the clinic till I reached home like a guardian angel became a dear presence. The drive on NH8 was the only reprieve for a craving mind—a mind that craved freedom from a shackled routine. No matter how much I tried to calm the roving heart which desired movies, lunches with friends, family celebrations and joyful time with my children, the turmoil would never leave.

I have seen NH8 in all its labour pains. The metamorphosis from a narrow, dusty and rutted path with listless bullock carts ambling along ignoring the other impatient travellers, to this present grand runway-like NH8, one of the best in India, has been dramatic. The diggings and the roadblocks for years which made me swear and stamp my feet, taught me many fine lessons in patience and acceptance! Endless waits at traffic signals on blazing afternoons when at times it would take seven to eight changes of the light for one's turn. There were times when a one-way journey to the clinic took me one and a half hours which meant I was on the road for over six hours, considering the two round trips. More poetry and more of this book took form on those days.

Monsoon season was the most challenging as the road to Kapashera became like a shallow lake overnight. On heavy rainy days one could see the cars stuck in at least two feet of water. The water covered the floor of the car and sitting tight in one's nicely polished shoes and ironed clothes, there wasn't anything much one could do except look in horror. It was probably sewage water from the surrounding, overflowing drains. One just had to numb one's mind regarding the origin of the water as the engine and the ignition both played truant and no amount of cursing or cajoling worked. The drivers desperately tried to revive their stalled engines with no success. Help came from the most unlikely quarters. A dozen or more beggar boys erupted like mushrooms, wading happily in the knee-deep lake. Barely eight or nine years old, they became car-towing and car-repair professionals. Their chests were bare as they made their way through the deep waters, trying to catch the eye of any stranded driver. One just had to flick a finger and a beggar boy would be by your side with a look and a smile that said: Here is the expert! Don't you worry!

The sight of a beggar boy at that point was like manna from the heavens. Each desperate motorist had just one prayer in his mind—'Oh please, I hope he comes to my car first'. These boys were at a premium as there were obviously more cars than beggars boys. They had learnt to start the engines by drying out the ignition, or whichever part of the car that got drenched by the rain, and they always delivered. They charged an absolutely fair amount which was according to the degree of distress the car driver exhibited on his face. Female drivers, of course, paid double the amount as they were obviously incapable of trudging through high waters in their sarees and high heels. Some adventurous men would roll up their trousers and try to tinker with the engine. Obviously their attempts were futile. It was some form of vehicle engineering that only those young boys had perfected. Besides the flooding, there were the treacherous puddles that became invisible once filled with murky water. They could be many feet deep. Only an experienced and trained eye could see what lay underneath the innocuous-looking puddle. If any car ran over even one of them, it was disastrous. The car had to be hauled from the deep crater, and it took four to five boys to lift it out of the deep ditch and put it on the road again.

To manoeuvre my car in all kinds of extreme weather and road conditions was my forte. It required more than dexterous driving skills. It required fine strategy. Father had taught me how to drive on a flooded road. The secret was never to release the accelerator and keep the clutch pressed hard and a lot of patience. I was one of those rare motorists who had memorised the measurement and placement of each crater to the nth degree and millimetre. This was simply because I manoeuvred them twice a day, every single day, in rain or shine. After all, practice does make one perfect. This got me through all thirty-eight monsoons, heavy squalls, dust storms, lightning, curfews, political unrest and all.

Over the years, NH8 became a living existence in my dull routine. It listened, it empathised and it befriended me in my loneliness. I developed a human relationship with my vehicle and my car became my safe space, haven and confidante. Over the decades, it has become more so. As life threw up unexpected complexities at various intervals, my car embraced me with unconditional loyalty as if we were in perfect mental and physical harmony. There were conversations and spirited discussions between the silent whirring of the car, NH8 and me. Difficult patients, school teachers, bad grades and difficult times, all were sorted out on NH8. I crafted complete chapters of this memoir during the two-hour commute, promising myself that I would note down each line as soon as I reached home. That was never to be! Yet the book stayed within the realms of my mind.

It was October 1984. Father and I had driven to the clinic in the morning as we always did. An old Hindi song filled us with a nostalgic well-being. Silently, we listened to the melancholic song. It was my father's favourite. As I mentioned earlier, once we left for the clinic, we were out of bounds for the entire world. There were no means to hear the daily news or what was happening in the city as it was pre-car radio times and there were no cell phones till the late nineties. It did not bother us for what we did not know, we did not miss.

As I sat in my clinic trying to finish the last few patients in the waiting room, there were murmurs outside. On enquiring, I heard people saying that something tragic had happened in the city. No one knew what the tragedy was. The air hung ominously pregnant with the stillness of impending danger. There was quietude all around.

Soon the last patient left. Father entered the clinic and said grimly, "Let's go a bit early today." Just a glance at his face and I suspected that something was not right. Quietly I sat in the car. Silently, we headed home as his look meant that he too didn't know the details. As we reached the highway, I saw black smoke arising from one of the farms on the right. Father, too, saw the smoke and his face became terse. I guessed there was a fire. I knew that a certain Mr Singh lived there with his two sons and their families.

"I know those people," he whispered, barely audible. He slowed down the car so we could have a better look. "They come to my clinic also, the two small children." I realised that we were whispering.

Father slowed the car further almost to a roll. This is when we caught sight of a huge mob running out of the farm. He reduced the speed and now the car was barely moving and we could see what was happening across the road. To my horror, I saw that the mob was carrying televisions, beds, fridges, boxes, washing machines and clothes piled on their heads. There must have been about twenty, thirty men running helter-skelter. All of them seemed to be in a hurry to get out. Some even had live chickens cackling away in panic, slung on their necks. It looked like a robbery or maybe vandalism.

Father parked the car on the muddy pathway and tried to

analyse the situation. We spotted a posse of policemen entering the farm and instructing those men. They seemed to be giving some orders. One of them looked as if he was in-charge and was gesticulating encouragingly. It was very clear that whatever was happening was in collusion with the police. Father understood the situation and his face looked even more grim. Within a few minutes the farm erupted in flames. The flames got higher by the second and the house burnt like tinder. Probably there were a lot of cut trees, wooden planks and gallons of oil stored for the generator as on all other farms. I saw the flames leaping high till the skies could bear them no longer.

The next moment, a strange smell wafted towards us and I inhaled it. It was like no other smell I had ever come across. I had smelled cadavers in the Anatomy classes and had survived the smell of burn wounds, putrid and decaying, in Kalawati and in Kapashera too. I had smelt blood in its various stages of putrefaction in the Obstetrics ward and it was revolting. I had never smelt the stench of burning flesh of living human beings. This smell permeates one's entire being and carves permanent fault lines in the mind. I never saw it happening yet the vision of the crying, struggling and pleading family overwhelmed me for years to come.

Never to be forgotten!

"Sahib, go away, it's dangerous. Don't park here!" I heard someone yell in a panic-stricken voice. I looked at the voice and recognised the gardener from the nearby nursery.

When we reached home, the TV blared the news that Prime Minister Indira Gandhi had been shot dead by her own guard. The guard happened to be a Sikh. Violence against Sikhs had been sparked off in the city. It had become uncontrollable like a conflagration, fanned by political motives. The mobs identified, killed and looted Sikhs randomly. It was a horrifying event.

Father had a few Sikh friends in the locality. As soon as he reached home, he rushed to their aid with rations and advised them to stay indoors for a couple of days.

The following day, what I feared and visualised had been proved right. The newspapers flashed headlines about Mr Singh's entire family that was tied to pillars and burnt alive, along with two children.

Every night, late at night, Father would tiptoe into his Sikh friend's home, his arms full of cartons of eggs, bread, milk and his words of assurance in his inimitable style. He did this for a couple of days till the mobs died down and peace was restored in the city.

It was one fine Saturday afternoon in 1993 and I was on my way back, driving at leisure because there was no need to hurry. The clinic had been peaceful with just the expected patients. No one had sprung a surprise. I was looking forward to spending a leisurely Saturday afternoon with the children. Maybe I would take them out for a nice lunch. There was a new outlet of McDonalds nearby. It was the first one in India. I had seen it in an American TV series and knew that it was a popular fast-food chain in America. The children had been waiting to go there as they had never had a burger from this chain before. It would be a good surprise for them and I knew they would love it. My husband would be back early too as it was a Saturday. With a song in my heart and a smile on my lips, I drove along. My daughter was three.

That day as I had left for the clinic, I sat for a while in my room and wrote a poem for my three-year-old daughter as she rode her new tricycle happily in the driveway. The sight of her joyous face as she sat on her red tricycle in a bright red sweater brought a lump in my throat.

"Mama, look, I can ride without holding it."

"Wow, you are awesome," I said absentmindedly, for my eyes were on my watch and my mind on my patients.

My son was busy making aeroplane swish sounds as he played with his favourite models on the porch. "Mama, mama, look; look there goes my plane," he said, his eyes shining like only an eight-year-old's can. Where did I have the time to stop and look at red bicycles and flying GI Joe planes?

I drove along the NH8 with thoughts of spending a lovely afternoon at McDonalds with my children. The road was not crowded, which was not unusual for a Saturday afternoon. I noticed random oil tankers spilling drops of oil from their overfilled tankers. The oil shone on the dark tarmac. There were the usual Saturday afternoon cars. After a moment or so, the skies darkened. Soon it started to drizzle and the rhythm of those little water droplets on my windscreen made me hum a favourite tune. The joy of the rain was short-lived. Suddenly, my car started to swerve and I could not keep it straight. No matter how much I tried, I could not control the steering wheel. The road was slippery and the tyres seemed to have no grip on the tarmac. I could see the car making zigzag, irregular patterns on the road, even though I had removed my foot from the accelerator. Trying to press the brakes gently made it swerve even more. I realised that this was it. With the morning memory of my children's faces, I prayed for them and said goodbye to all who were precious in my life. I felt Father's arm around me and he held me against him as if to save me from the injuries.

There was a ditch about ten feet deep on both sides of the road. I was told later by the passers-by, some of whom were my patients, that my car had turned turtle and landed in that ditch. When I opened my eyes, I was sitting in the front seat of a strange car and the man beside me was speeding maniacally down the road, blowing the horn like the alarm of an ambulance. I studied his face and concluded that he looked reliable.

I knew I was injured when I felt some fluid flowing down my face. As I ran my fingers to wipe away those streaks, I realised that it was blood. I could feel that my clothes were soaked in blood and clung to me. I took stock of my vital signs; my pulse was racing as fast as this stranger drove. The bleeding continued, although the dripping blood seemed to have reduced. Must have formed clots, I assumed. As I ran my hand over my face again I withdrew it fast as all I felt were sharp glass splinters on my scalp and face.

I could see, I could hear and I could think. That was reassuring!

I handed the stranger my handbag.

"My phone number is...please call up my home in case I lose consciousness," I blabbered quickly.

With the amount of blood dripping from my head, passing out was imminent.

This angel took me to the Emergency of Wellington Hospital, a government tertiary care hospital. After the necessary paperwork, I was given a bed where I lay shivering. Soon a puddle of blood formed beneath me on the sheetless steel bed. It was the first time I noticed the condition of government hospitals from a patient's perspective.

The stranger who had driven me to the Emergency had gone to look for a phone booth to make the phone calls to the numbers I had provided. Those were the pre-cellphone days. My mother-in-law was home. There were many callers that afternoon. Some were my patients who had seen my car in the ditch. "There is a woman in a red sweater in a blue car; is it the lady doctor of Kapashera?" they asked her. She did not remember the colour of the saree or the red sweater I had worn that morning, so I could not be identified on the phone, and the woman in the red sweater remained a mystery for the time being. The blue colour of the car matched. She tried calling my husband in the hospital where he worked, but he had already left the hospital and could not be reached.

Panic-stricken, she called my brother who had an office near the hospital. Luckily, he answered the phone and reached the hospital in fifteen minutes. I still remember his shocked expression when he saw my condition. There was little he managed to do or could do but the concern on his face was strangely reassuring. The stranger who had driven me seemed to be the most efficient, as he brought in a nurse and a junior resident to have a look at my injuries.

The nurse came, peeped in and went away.

"I am feeling very cold. Please give me a blanket," I said in the loudest voice I could manage but it came out as a squeak. Her back was already out of the door and had retreated too far to hear. I did not get a blanket.

She returned and looked busy—busy with just walking around and trying not to look at me. She hadn't even examined my wounds in the thirty minutes I had been on that bed.

I whimpered again, "My leg is paining; please give me an

injection for the pain."

She looked at me and left the room again.

Why is she even coming in? I wondered.

A short while after the nurse left, a young enthusiastic-looking doctor, probably on his first duty in Emergency, entered. I tried to catch his attention by playing the doctor card.

"I am a doctor. My husband is a surgeon. Please have a look at my injuries."

"Of course we will, you just keep lying down quietly," he said in a familiar, patronising tone. It sounded like the one I used for illiterate villagers. I was surely getting tit for tat. I was sure that I would never ignore any of my patients if they asked for a blanket.

As I lay on the narrow hospital bed, bleeding, in pain and shivering, I learnt the biggest lesson of my life. I learnt the finest nuances of compassionate patient care in that one hour.

My brother kept looking aghast. There was not much he could do anyway. He tried but was not of much help in getting me a doctor or even a blanket. I had come to the hospital at two pm, soaked in my own blood, cold and shivering. Even after two hours, I didn't have a blanket or a painkiller; and this was one of the biggest hospitals in Delhi!

My husband finally entered with hurried steps at four pm with the stoicism and the intent look of a surgeon. His unrelenting expression, annoying at times, was effective in hospitals, restaurants, grocery stores and even in primary schools and, of course, the office of the Principal. I had seen this first-hand and speak from deep experience. The look could intimidate people, especially teachers and doctors. He got his way most of the time. I knew things would move now. Just a few seconds more and the nurse would get a dressing down. I waited with sadistic pleasure.

Suddenly things started to move. I didn't hear him utter a single word, yet the nurse came rushing with a new red blanket still in its plastic packet. It was obvious it was a brand new one and had not been used by any other patient.

The senior resident had lost his fake confident look and now looked apologetic. He tried to say something meaningful, but all he could stutter was, "Sir, Sir." The snooty nurse, the senior resident and the junior rookie, all got to work, guided by my husband. Peeping diligently at my forehead to assess the damage, the junior rookie was relegated to handing cotton swabs to clean up the rivulets of dried blood from my face. The stitching tray had been set up and the senior resident was ready to begin. The glass splinters were removed from my face. The cuts and wounds were stitched with quick, adept stitches—as adept as they could be in the given circumstances. I could sense the disagreement and disapproval on my husband's face at the quality of the stitches but he couldn't do much. There was no way he would take matters in his hands as treating one's own relatives was a big 'no' in the medical circles.

Once the wound was stitched and bandaged, and I was ready to leave, we searched around for the kind stranger who had brought me to the hospital. We found him waiting in the corridor. He told us the exact sequence of events that had landed me and my car into the ditch because his car was just behind mine. He saw my vehicle pirouette on the road several times before it turned turtle and fell into the ditch ten feet below.

"I could not open the car doors as they were jammed and had to pull you out from the windscreen," he said. His wife had originally been in the front, but she moved to the back to allow me more room. I remembered telling him that the blood dripping from my head would stain and spoil his car seats.

We thanked him profusely and took his address and intended to visit him with an appropriate token of gratitude.

Back home in the late evening, one of my husband's colleagues, a plastic surgeon, visited us. He was horrified at the sight of the shoddy stitching that had been done all over my forehead. Looking at the expressions on his face, I figured that I must look really unsightly. "No way, no way," he kept muttering.

Immediately he took us to Lok Nayak Hospital, my husband's hospital. They rushed me into the OT and removed those crude stitches. I was given seventy proper stitches that were a work of art. The surgeon examined his handiwork and beamed with pride.

"You won't be able to see a single mark in a few months. It was good that we opened them up," he said. With all the pain and distress of a major accident, a few marks on my face was the last thing to bother me.

"Oh, there were many glass splinters still embedded deep inside," he added, looking at my face. "I took them all out."

CHAPTER SIXTEEN

Bijwasan and the Harvest Season

IT WAS MAINLY the Bijwasan folks who were landowners. There were big landowners and small ones. The big ones owned sprawling fields that rolled away for acres into the horizon. The small ones had only a couple of hectares. This was green, productive land with plenty of groundwater resources and abundance of sunlight all year around. The landowners grew wheat, with a few vegetables spread on the rows of soil mounds criss-crossing the fields. A few ambitious ones sowed rice. Pulses were common along with mustard. Mustard fields were the prettiest as the yellow flowers shone so bright in the winter sun and were a generous source of mustard greens, mustard oil and mustard seeds. The oil was extracted not by any machines but an ox cart that went around the mill. The dregs after extracting the oil were put in the cattle feed. Every part of the crop was put to use. The farmers sold the vegetables in the local markets and kept the green leaves and inedible parts to be used as green fodder. Mixed with dry hay, it became the ideal food for their animals.

Most of the homes in Bijwasan had a cow or a buffalo and a rare sheep. The cows and the buffaloes were used only for milk and were treated like family members. When the cows were without milk, the family would wait a year until they birthed a calf and became productive again. No one resented their consumption of fodder. Young calves were fed before the cows were milked. Since this was a vegetarian community, no cattle were slaughtered for meat. The bulls were used to pull carts, plough the land, and to run the mill to extract mustard oil while the others were used to draw water from wells. No one was ever in a hurry to discard animals that had become unproductive. The farmers simply retired the animal who then lazed in the sun all day chewing cud. They waited for the animal to pass away naturally. I witnessed an inherent sense of affection when these people mentioned their cows. I know of a family who told me that if their cow was sick, the whole family would go without food till she started to eat. As a result, hormone injections to boost milk supply were unheard of in the eighties and nineties; milk-boosting injections and greed came around the 2000s when India got its taste of globalisation.

Liberal spending patterns gave rise to a liberal need for money. Money had to be earned, whichever way. Everyone wanted more milk, more vegetables, and more wheat so they could make more money. Hormone injections, growth chemicals, genetically-modified seeds and harmful fertilisers flooded the markets.

There were a few vets around, but like the quacks they injected steroids and a painkiller for every sickness so the farmers avoided them. They fed their cows well and made sure they raised 'happy' cows. It was rare that cows fell sick.

If one ever fell sick and died, it was accepted as God's will and mourned for exactly the same period as they would a family member.

When I look back, it seemed like a utopian world where no evil existed.

Milk was like oil for an engine. It made the world go round. The family kept most of the milk for consumption and it was distributed to the whole clan according to their specific needs. The pregnant women and growing children got a larger share while the men were given the amounts they desired; the remaining milk was divided amongst the girls and the women of the household. Everyone had to follow this rationing protocol and no one complained as there was plenty of milk to go around, and plenty was left over which was to be poured into clay pots to be churned into butter. An extremely important task. The butter, too, had its rationing. Some members of the family were butter lovers and ate spoonfuls of it with the rice and lentils while the rest of the butter was bartered to neighbours in exchange for green vegetables, rice, sugar or some tailoring jobs. The leftover butter was put on the fire to make ghee.

Ghee was a measure of the happiness index of the family. With ghee, families could make laddoos, halva and other sweets. It was collected to send to the married daughters and was a status symbol and marked the well-being of a family.

When a daughter-in-law had a baby, the female neighbours would jest and ask her, "How many kilos of ghee has your mother sent for you?" It was obviously her mother's task to present this precious commodity to the in-laws, especially if it was a boy. The mother would visit her daughter with at least fifteen kg of ghee, a year's supply of baby clothes and toys, and complete outfits for every member of the in-laws family. The birth of a girl didn't require much ghee or jubilation. The amount of ghee a new mother received from her parents ensured the respect and status that she would get in her marital home. If the girl's family had no cattle of their own, the poor mother had no choice but to buy it from retail. The neighbourly women would click their tongues in a show of disapproval and pity.

In the eighties, the nineties, and well into the 2000s, despite rich buffalo milk and a ghee diet, none of my patients ever suffered from Cardiac disease or Hypertension. Not one patient back then had a fatty liver. There were no gyms, no fad diets, and no statins; and I do not remember prescribing any antihypertensives or cholesterol-lowering drugs to anyone in the first half of my career. The distance they walked every single day to work in the fields, to collect green fodder, dung, and clean huge homesteads, most likely kept them healthy in the long run. The women worked almost ten hours a day with short breaks to feed the baby and cook meals. I never heard of anyone mentioning an afternoon siesta.

Today, eighty percent of both men and women come with fatty livers and high cholesterol. The diets are the same but with all the fields being sold, there is no place left to walk to. I relentlessly educated them about the benefits of milk over ghee and thankfully, most of them learnt and practised what I taught.

It was a feast for the eyes to see the graceful women of Bijwasan walking to their farms, their white skirts flowing like clouds and their dupattas, bright and colourful, billowing against the clear skies—shades of red, green, orange and royal blue flashing in the sun. These dupattas always had an edging of a silver lace to complement the delightful colours. The width and intricacy of the edging was a sign of the social status of the lady. These women were tall and lithe which made them look stunning in the blouses they wore a few inches away from the waist. They would stroll through the fields with stacks of hay on their heads. One hand would hold the green fodder and the other would be swinging by their side. The balancing act, as they manoeuvred precariously along the narrow pathways in the fields with the heavy fodder on their heads, imparted the characteristic sway to the narrow waists they all had.

I saw these women come to Father's farm every morning, armed with a sickle to cut, and a cloth bag to collect the green grass for their cattle. It was a symbiotic arrangement that saved Father the trouble of getting the lawns mowed, and the women got the green fodder they needed. I enjoyed looking at them working their scythes in rhythmic motion. It was an idyllic setting. By noon, these women would have collected as much as they needed and could be seen carrying huge bundles of grass on their heads. Collecting green, freshly-cut grass was a daily activity that had no social divide. The rich and poor women all did it. I, obviously, missed some links of this idyllic setting. Somewhere, some women were unhappy and I came to know of their sadness later when I heard of the suicides on the railway tracks. I learnt that there is always a dichotomy in every life situation, even in places that seem perfect.

Some days the women managed to hitch a ride in their husband's or neighbour's tractor.

The tractor was the lifeline of these farmers. Those who didn't own one, dreamt of buying it as the ultimate dream, and those who owned them were the envy of the rest. These hardy machines were used to plough the fields and get them ready for the next sowing. Most importantly, the tractors ferried the tonnes of golden wheat to the wholesale *mandis* for the auctions. The only vehicle they had was the family tractor which sufficed for most travelling needs which included visits to the doctor, attending family weddings, and ferrying the bride to the groom's home. The tractors became the hearse, the ambulance, a night shelter, election vehicles and much more. They could be dressed up or down.

These women started to come directly from the fields to the clinic, and opened their small *potlis, (*cloth bags) of freshly-plucked spinach, mustard leaves, verdant coriander, fenugreek greens and sparkling white radishes right on my table with love and pride. My table would look like a vegetable market but I never took offence for this act of affection.

"I got this for you," they would say, hoping to see my eyes shine with pleasure, and they did. "Oh, beautiful, it's just what I wanted today!" I would smile back and say with heartfelt joy. The love I developed for fresh, leafy vegetables, because of these women, has lasted me a lifetime. On some days the women came to visit me with a steel container full of freshly-churned buttermilk.

"It's fresh. I took it out for you," one of them would say happily. I could see that she would be panting and out of breath. Obviously she had walked from Bijwasan to my clinic in the blistering heat of June.

Life was busy for these simple people. The large farms required hard labour all round the year. Making dung cakes was a year-round activity. The women would collect cow dung and make igloo-like structures that dotted the entire rural skyline; these were used to store the hay for the cattle. The cow dung huts were as water repellent as anything could ever be as I never saw any cement being used to make them watertight. Hundreds of dung cakes had to be patted into round pancakes and plastered on the walls to dry. The dried dung cakes were then collected to be stored. Dung cakes might sound strange, but they were the primary fuel to keep the home fires burning as there were no gas lines or compressed gas till the 2000s. The new brides had to accept the mantle of the official dung-cake maker along with the mother-in-law. Some quietly accepted this chore as a part of marriage, but others had delicate sensitivities, so they refused. The ones who refused were the unhappiest lot, as they were the outliers and came to me with various real or imagined ailments.

It was the mother-in-law who was, invariably, the supreme force in the family, and I learnt gradually that if I had to get anywhere with any patient, I had to be in her good books. If a patient had to visit me again to complete a course for any ailment, it was my job to impress upon the mother-in-law and convince her that in the long run, the problem may give trouble. Conviction, cajoling, compliments and reasoning, all came in useful.

Along with getting fodder and making dung cakes, the women had to clean up the large houses, start the kitchen fires, cook, wash the clothes and feed the babies, and do a few other chores which were women-centric. With the women managing the home fires and the children, the men had to buy the seeds, chop the fodder and bathe the sick cattle every day. They had their first meal of the day after they finished feeding and bathing the cattle, and walking around the farmland looking for any weeds or infestations of germs.

Milking of the cows was gender neutral in most homes. Milking was also according to the preference of the cow. The cattle had preferences as to who could milk them.

"I can't visit my parents ever," a lady said.

"Why?"

"My cow doesn't let anyone else milk her," she said matter-of-factly. Their lives were strung around their cattle as they fell sick if not milked.

The harvest season took its toll as it meant an added workload to an already bustling lifestyle, yet it was welcomed with a charming joie de vivre. The harvest was called *Lavani* in the local lingo, a charming word. During this season, the entire family got to work. Every member of the family had to pitch in. Division of labour was according to the physical capabilities. There was no gender discrimination, no age bias and no socioeconomic bias. The old and the pregnant women stayed at home and contributed their bit. The very old and infirm sat on their charpoys and churned butter, made ghee, chopped the greens and minded the children. The pregnant and young unmarried girls cooked and kept the meals ready for the men and women as they returned exhausted and sunburnt from the fields. Sometimes they even carried the food in steel tiffins to the fields. Men and women put in equal hours of work and enjoyed the reapings equally.

Once the grain was ripe in the fields, it became a race against time as the crop had to be cut at absolutely the right time. If even one cloud showed up, the cutting went on all through the night. To have golden wheat sheaves soaked in rain was a constant nightmare for all the farmers. The bigger farmers could afford to hire labourers during harvest time to do the cutting and making sheaves of wheat. After the golden grain was collected, the older, more experienced men were relegated the task of going to the wholesale market to negotiate the best rates for their labour. Even a gain of one rupee per kilo was a cause for celebration as the sacks carried the wheat in tonnes.

Besides the golden kernels of wheat, there were other things that were a fallout bonus. The hay! It had to be collected and dried and chopped to be used as cattle fodder for rainy weather and stored in makeshift cow dung huts and concrete storage rooms. The strong youngsters would make bales of hay, load them on the tractors to take them to the chopping machine, chop the bales into perfect-size fodder and then take them to the designated storage area. The hay-baling was extremely back-breaking work, yet no one minded doing it as it meant having a constant supply of fodder for the cattle for the whole year. Although the hay could be cut two or three times a year, the harvest yield was the best. The best hay had its own specifications. There could be no moisture in it as that would cause rotting, so it was raked and left in the sun to dry for a few days. The size of the chopped hay had to be small so the cattle were able to chew.

The men operated the tractors, got the sheaves of the grain and put them in the threshers to be thrashed into pearls of golden wheat separating them from the chaff. The sheaves had to be put right inside the machines with the whole arm. This was the era before the automatic machines had made their appearance. Obviously, the ruthless blade did not distinguish between human and botanical matter. Accidents happened and were usually frightful as the blades of the machine were sharp. Many patients visited me with sliced fingers, chopped hands and limbs. A few times, some young men had their entire arm hacked off by the machine. In fact, every village had a sizeable number of men with just one arm and they carried their remaining arm with pride, as a soldier would. There was no shame as this was considered an accident of valour.

Once, one of these ill-starred guys came to visit me in my clinic. He walked in with another young male, both of whom strode in with an assumed confidence to ward off the pain. Here was this young man carrying his limb in a towel. He did not wince or whimper even once.

"Please manage this," said his aide, without an ounce of doubt about my skills in stitching up limbs wrapped in towels.

"What…I don't do this; my clinic is not equipped for such large operations." I recoiled at the sight of the freshly-chopped limb still oozing blood.

"You did my brother's finger," the aide said, "that's why I came to you."

"No, no, take him to the hospital," I said. "I can do the first aid to stop the bleeding, but take him to Safdarjung Hospital. They will do a good job." I knew I should not be attaching chopped limbs.

Luckily, there were no arguments. The armless man sat stoically while I administered first aid and gave him an injection for pain and soon enough, I saw him off to Safdarjung Hospital.

My confidence increased with stitching wounds and cuts of all sizes and shapes. I knew that if I refused to stitch up a patient, they would just go home and wait for it to heal on its own; most would not go to hospital.

I had not yet ventured into detached body parts. There were lacerated wounds and infected ones; wounds that had no shape and wounds that wouldn't stop bleeding. How could anyone stitch them? They had no edges. I saw them all and tried my best to stitch them with confidence laced with nervousness.

There was Sonu, who refused to go to the hospital. In those days, people feared hospitals because they were strange and unknown places. Anyway, this lad of twenty-something had cut his index finger in the hay machine. As he unwrapped the blood-soaked cloth from his hand, I saw that a thin tissue had kept his finger attached to the bone. It hung and dangled loosely. I knew nothing about hand surgery. This was a lacerated wound with uneven skin tags ready to fall off.

"I'm sorry but you must go to the hospital, I can't do this," I said resolutely.

"I am not going to any hospital," he argued. "I will just go home and let it heal on its own."

He got up to leave, but before he exited the room he turned back to me.

"Either you do whatever you can do, or God will help me."

I looked at his mother, who nodded in agreement. Convinced by their conviction, I got the tray, suture material, curved needle and swabs.

I admit that I lacked the sophisticated machinery they had in hospitals, but I was proud of my stitching set and knew that I had the best suture material available in the country, thanks to the surgeon at home. He made sure I had the best self-dissolving catgut, top-class curved needles, the sharpest forceps and stacks of sterile gauze. Sterile gauze and Sofia Tulle were a real luxury in the eighties and nineties because no one had seen or heard of them. They were extremely expensive yet I had an ample supply of them. When the tools are right, the job at hand gives immense joy. So was the case with stitching procedures that I undertook in my clinic and worked on them as an artist. The cost of the materials I used far exceeded the payment I received for my services. Yet, it never bothered me as I was immensely proud of my procedures.

I washed Sonu's wound thoroughly with saline and the picture became clearer. The more I examined the finger, the more aghast I was at its hopeless state. I knew I could be making a grave mistake. I carefully aligned the finger and slowly worked my way around, stitching it neatly, tag by tag until all the skin tags were joined together. It looked well done and complete. Patience was the key. I had that in plenty. After my artistic stitching, the finger looked fine to me from the outside and the patient looked satisfied with my prowess. Only I knew that the blood vessels and nerves that may have got injured inside, were still lying unstitched. Anyway, keeping a masked face, I prayed for his recovery and looked at the boy's face for any trace of distress.

The fear of Sonu developing gangrene haunted me for a week till I could see definitive signs of healing. I warned his family that he had to visit me daily for a new dressing or I would have to send him to the hospital if the finger changed colour.

In seven days, the finger was nice and pink and displayed movement and signs of life. The family said they always knew it would heal. It was obvious, they said, as I gave a weak smile.

The moment a doctor picks up her instruments, no one doubts her skills. The patient is confident that nothing will go wrong and the doctor is confident in her ability or she would never pick up her tools.

The shadow of doubt in her mind is cast only by the fear of the patient's reactions in case things go wrong.

The fear of unimaginable consequences of my actions

dogged me every time. Despite my misgivings about stitching big wounds, I worked on plenty of injured limbs. Often faced with limbs that had been caught in a running fan, industrial cutters, kitchen knives, doorways and blades of all kinds, I had no option but to stitch-up.

Whenever the patients from Bijwasan dwindled, I knew that it must be the harvest season because everything was put on hold for the harvest. March and April were very lean seasons for me, but the patients would return as April marched its way out. If I called a pregnant patient in for a check-up, she would reply, "I can't come. Who will come with me? My husband is in the fields." Children were neglected, too. If a child was very sick, the grandmothers who were holding the fort at home would be forced to trudge in at times. "I had to walk all the way," she would plead breathlessly. "He is very sick," holding the child towards me. They just could not afford to neglect the crops and their cattle. If I chided a patient for leaving the course of antibiotics incomplete, she would simply say, "It's harvest time, how could I come?" I understood.

Soon after the harvest, the women who came in would be a few pounds leaner, with sunburnt faces due to working in the blazing heat all day long, yet they looked content. They bought new clothes, arranged weddings, and there was a general atmosphere of jubilation. Glowing with the exuberance of a job well done, some handed me an envelope shyly that held the wedding card and said, "I am getting married. Please come." These were the happy moments that provided me with untiring reasons to continue my practice.

CHAPTER SEVENTEEN

Mornings at the Railway Track

A RAILWAY LINE passed through Bijwasan. It was the custom that the women would gather outside their houses in the early hours of the morning, coalesce into smaller groups and make their way to the fields which lay on either side of the railway track.

A strange fact about India and a few other Asian countries is that the railway tracks form an integral part of daily lives. They are the first choice of venue for many personal needs and normal activities of life. Some places even have complete vegetable markets right on the track. Clothes can be seen fluttering on makeshift lines by the tracks. Babies sleep in cloth hammocks while their mothers stir the cooking pots over wood fires. The moment the whistle of the train in the distance is heard, the wares and babies are gathered till the train passes by and life resumes till the next whistle.

Groups of five or six people could sit in a row on the track and chit-chat during the mundane job. What an ingenuous way to develop camaraderie and oneness!

The ritual of outdoor defecation was not a financial limitation as most of them were very wealthy farmers. It was a way of life. The men exchanged the daily news, political turmoil, land prices and the latest procuring rates of wheat; while the women giggled and whispered little stories about the mothers-in-law, their children, husbands, upcoming festivals and the gifts they may or may not receive. In fact, everything under the sun was ripped apart and discussed amidst giggles and tears. Soon all the notes that had to be exchanged were exchanged, the main jobs were done and the women would happily make their way home to their cattle, husbands and the rest of their demanding family chores; and the day ahead seemed survivable.

The daily meets on the railway track were no less effective than a therapist's couch.

Under the shine of the camaraderie lay a dark side. An ugly reality. I heard it said casually from my staff and some patients. "Women are found lying dead on the tracks every day," they said.

An older woman from Bijwasan willingly shared the details of the suicides that happened routinely on the railway tracks.

"We see two or three of them every day," she said in a whisper.

"Why are women found dead every single day on the railway tracks?"

"Some young brides are thrown on the tracks by their mothers-in-law."

They were probably egged on by the husband and his sisters for her not getting enough dowry or producing a son. Dowry was one of the biggest reasons for pushing them to suicide. They were taunted and locked up in a room without food or water for days on end.

Not producing a son was the next worst thing. The new mother would not be given food and not allowed to breastfeed. I know of a few women who were subjected to multiple forced abortions if the ultrasound indicated a female foetus. Some came to me with tear-stained faces, anaemic and starved, with a history of having seven to eight abortions. I came across a patient who told me that her mother-in-law would kick her in the abdomen when she feared that another girl was on the way.

What would a young woman do when subjected to abuses like:

> *"You witch,"*
> *"You good for nothing whore,"*
> *"Go hang yourself,"*
> *"You go drown yourself,"*
> *"You girl-bearing wretch."*

What could these unhappy women do? The parents could not and would not take them back.

There comes a time in everyone's lives when one says '*enough is enough.*'

They would make their way to the tracks in silence, tiptoeing out of their homes with heavy hearts, leaving their husbands and children sleeping. The dark, shadowy figures stepped out into the ignominy of the early morning before the sunrise made them weak in their resolve. They covered their faces with their dupattas and lay in anonymity and anticipation on the cold steel tracks, waiting. It was convenient. The blackness of the night embraced them silently as they waited for the rumbling train in the distance. I heard that these suicides were not incidental but took place on a daily basis.

The bodies were identified and cremated and the last rites performed in hushed silence. Her parents would be informed a day or two after the cremation and told that their daughter had died of natural causes. At times a heart attack was stated to be the cause of death. No one asked any questions and no one wondered about the probability of a heart attack in a twenty-year-old.

No one ever talked about whose daughter or daughter-in-law it was for even if they knew her identity, people remained silent. They were like brothers-in-arms because they had grown up and lived together for generations and shared the same beliefs. Everyone in the village knew this was happening, but no reports were filed with the police. There were no doctors to question the cause of death, no investigations, no questions whatsoever, and no one in the village dared to open their mouths for fear of being ousted from the community.

I envisioned one sad, lonely woman whispering in the evening to her neighbour that she would not return home the next morning. I wondered if….

She took many months to decide?
Or did she make the decision that very night?
Did she share her woes with her friends?
Did she call up her brothers?
Did she talk to her mother?
Did she take this step in a fit of anger?
Or was it resignation?
Did she want to get up and run from the track?

Digging deep, I heard that some women were even killed

at home by suffocations, starvations or poisoning and their bodies were thrown on the tracks in the morning so they wouldn't be recognised. Their dead bodies would be declared as unidentified and cremated by the police.

Although these suicides and murders sound barbaric, the railway line seemed the best and the least painful option.

"Some daughters are killed too," continued my superb raconteur Ramrati, quite content to see my scandalised look. I nodded my head at intervals so she wouldn't stop.

"Why daughters?" I asked.

"When daughters go out and meet boys from another caste or community," began the wise Ramrati, "they have to die."

"Why?" I exclaimed.

"Honour killing. The girl's father and brother lose face if she is allowed to live."

A middle-aged farmer from Bijwasan was a regular at my clinic. It was obvious that Ram Swaroop was a landowner. One day he came in with a headache, "Please can you check my blood pressure?" he said.

I took the BP apparatus and quietly measured his blood pressure.

"A bit on the high side," I said. "What's the matter?" I sensed that the problem was not the blood pressure but something else on his mind.

"It's my daughter,"

"What happened to her?"

"I found her with the neighbour's son."

"That's okay, just let her be," I tried to calm him. "It happens, times are changing."

Ram Swaroop got agitated. "What do you know of family

honour?" His face contorted in pain and agony. "She is my favourite child."

I listened quietly for a moment. I knew that if I said anything he could get inflamed.

He sat quietly with his face left loose, expressionless. A few moments passed in silence, then he muttered, "She will have to die." I shuddered. "What, you will kill her?"

"Yes, there is no other way to save face." I could see he was fighting his own battles within him. "The whole village will laugh at me if I don't."

Days later, a patient from Bijwasan told me that a young girl was found dead in her home. People wondered what happened. The death of the young girl was passed off as Voodoo.

No one in the urban world knew of these murders and honour killings.

Things started to look up in the 2000s when there was a paradigm shift in power for women. Legally, the women started receiving their fair share in the father's property. The Indian courts had come full circle and most of the rulings in domestic violence were in favour of the women.

CHAPTER EIGHTEEN

The People of Rajokri

WHILE BIJWASAN WAS blessed with vast, cultivable land, a small village called Rajokri sat on the other side of the highway. It had stone crushers that made sand dust all day and night long. Its air was cloudy with the stone dust. It took almost half an hour to walk from the village to my clinic. No one owned tractors in Rajokri for there were no farmers. The rich people owned bullock carts pulled by a buffalo; others had bicycles. The majority of the people who came to me from Rajokri were labourers who worked at the stone crushers. The rich contractors owned motorcycles and cars. A few years later, in the nineties, most had bicycles, and the older ones preferred to hire cycle and autorickshaws that had started plying between Rajokri and Kapashera. These patients had to be seen before everyone else, or they might have to pay the rickshaw man extra money for the waiting time. The other patients waiting for their turn understood and never created a fuss, for they knew that the rickshaw man had to take his passenger back and might even leave the poor patient fretting in the May heat.

Summer months were the worst as the patients would trudge into my clinic dripping sweat. The mothers would wrap up the children in layers of cloth to protect them from sunstrokes. As they entered the clinic they would stand in front of the water cooler and take deep, relaxed breaths as the cool air touched their sweat-soaked bodies. They would sigh in relief as they gulped bottles of chilled water which were kept in abundance on the tables in the waiting room. In the earlier decade before I acquired a fridge, I had a clay pot called *ghada* to provide the cold water. It was in the late nineties that I got around to buying a fridge. It was a novelty for the patients as access to this luxury, in my neck of the woods, was not a reality till the 2000s.

I learnt to recognise the patients who came from Rajokri because their clothes were a tad crumpled and not as bright or new as the Bijwasan folks. Their complexion was also darker. I found it both strange and interesting that just a few kilometres could give rise to such distinct dialects and appearances.

Bijwasan was the land of plenty where people owned land, cattle and had their own homes, while Rajokri was a small village that housed a few farmers and mostly contractors and labourers. The village was known for the numerous stone crushers that made cement and gravel. The sand and gravel for construction work in Delhi and neighbouring states was supplied by this village, so the need for cheap labour was perpetual. With so much need it was natural that hordes of immigrants from Uttar Pradesh and Bihar made their way to Rajokri. This is when the entity 'urban slums' became a reality. These labourers travelled long distances crouching in overcrowded trains to reach Delhi in the hope of jobs. I found it sad that these young men could never have imagined the life they were heading to, that began and ended with breaking stones; then lifting and loading them onto the waiting trucks, with the eagle-eyed contractor timing every movement and tracking every lost second.

Seven or eight of the labourers rented one small room and pooled in the rent and groceries, cooking simple one-pot meals to save enough to send a large part of their wages home to their families. The concept or choice of a bed or a toilet wasn't available to anyone back then. They slept on the floor and relieved themselves on the barren land which was aplenty in Rajokri.

The contractors were paid well by the construction mafia. They employed labourers and paid them on a daily basis. These daily-wagers always lived a hand-to-mouth existence; their jobs were not secure as the payment was on a daily basis and they were fired over minor things.

It was the contractors who made all the cash.

I was getting both the contractors and the labourers as patients. The contractors came by in their latest cars, clad in a white shirt and white pants. The bulge of the pot belly was constrained under a flashy black belt. The dark sunglasses were a sign of wealth, so they all sported the flashiest ones along with pointed white shoes that reminded me of Bollywood heroes. The most prominent memory I have of these contractors is of the fat wad of notes they dug out from their deep pockets when they had to pay me. "How much is the bill?" Ram Swaroop, a regular patient asked.

"150 rupees," was the usual reply. Ram Swaroop counted the money and handed it to my staff. Once, he made the audacious mistake to say to my staff, "Keep the change." I was outraged!

"This is a clinic not a charity bowl," I said sharply. His face fell. I could tell that he knew no better. He did not flash his money to insult us; it was just the way he was.

In the years that followed, Ram Swaroop became the most courteous of them all and would bring in a regular flow of injured labourers. I developed a certain respect for him as he acquiesced to my request to pay one month extra wages to the injured men. This small step for the labourers changed their lives. In fact, he convinced more contractors to do the same. He covered the entire cost of the treatment and even offered them some extra money for food. It was a win-win situation. The labourers didn't feel exploited and the contractors were free of the constant fear nagging at them that the labourers might go to the police or the labour union.

Rajokri was one of the villages with no infrastructure at all. There were no sewage lines, no drains, no potable water and no medical facilities. The makeshift drains lay open, buzzing with flies. The pipes were rotting in places and the sewage water contaminated the drinking water. I had never set foot in any of the villages, but I could guess the lack of infrastructure in the village, with patients filling in the gaps in my information. Disease patterns were in tandem with the missing facilities in the village. Bijwasan, which had a reasonable sewage system and substantial potable water was free from the big three—typhoid, jaundice and gastroenteritis, all water-borne diseases. The disease pattern of this village was easy to gather for it was typical and wasn't complicated like that of Bijwasan. The latter, with its evolved lifestyle, was fraught with many social and psychological discords. When living is so primordial, how can the ailments be complicated?

Living in crowded rooms caused an easy spread of disease. If one person came to my clinic with typhoid, another with the same disease would visit the next day, then another, and then another until all the roommates were infected with typhoid or jaundice. There was no way I could tell them to stop sharing meals as that was the basis of their existence. Eight or more roommates ate in one plate with their hands; they did not have the means to buy two or more plates or spoons.

In the eighties and nineties, the only cases I received were complicated ones of typhoid. In the broiling summer months, I had at least five IV lines running in the inside room. A few children with consistent vomiting lay in the waiting room for observation; the rest of the patients would be fever cases who needed ice packs.

Along with these big three of typhoid, jaundice and gastroenteritis, tuberculosis constituted the major spectrum of Rajokri illnesses. How could I treat them successfully when there was an impediment to treating these simple illnesses? The quacks. The hundreds of the omnipresent quacks who weren't qualified to treat anyone made things very difficult. Only a very small percentage of patients came to me in the initial stages. Most of them eventually came after days of detrimental treatment from these quacks. The children with gastroenteritis would arrive in a moribund state and I was left to pick up the pieces. I suspect that when the quack feared that the child would die, he quickly referred him to me just to save his own skin. The mothers carried their little infants with gloomy expressions and stared at me with panic-stricken, helpless and desperate faces which haunted me for days. Years later, I painted these faces on canvas to express the images and the feelings they conjured in my mind.

Do I regret gazing at my patients to seek what lay behind those eyes?

Was it wrong to make my patients the muse for my art?

"Please please, save my child," a mother begged as if I could reverse the child's sickness instantly. One look and I knew that the child dangled precariously between life and death. Wrinkled skin on the abdomen, sunken eyes, sunken head, and a limp body, I dreaded those patients. "Why didn't you come yesterday?" I would ask a bit irked as I looked accusingly at the mother.

"We went to the doctor nearby," was the usual reply. "Today, he told us to bring the child here," they would answer in the hope and the belief that all would be okay once the child entered my clinic. Families who brought their children to me after a lack of success with the quacks scared me. My treatment worked most of the time but what if one day, it didn't? I knew that if I couldn't save even one child, it would take just a breath to change this deference to vindictiveness.

With a prayer on my lips and hope in my heart, I worked on these sick children and watched in relief as the grateful parents left the clinic.

One day, a contractor came into my clinic in his brand new car. He was in the usual contractor attire of white pants, white shirt and pointed shoes, and his deportment conveyed a sense of importance. He was followed by two labourers who carried a thin, waif-like labourer who seemed unconscious. One look at the injured man's face and I knew that he could not be a day older than nineteen.

"Please take a look at him," said the flashy-looking contractor in an authoritative tone. He hadn't bothered to remove his goggles.

"Please take off your goggles." I was annoyed at this hint of arrogance. He obliged and looked appropriately respectful.

"How did he get hurt?"

"A load of gravel fell on his head," he said.

"How heavy was it?" I noticed that the young, injured labourer was wincing in pain at every breath. I examined him and ruled out a fracture of the ribs. The cervical region seemed okay too.

"About fifty kilos," said one of the labourers who had initially carried the guy into my clinic.

"No, no, it was about fifteen kilos," said the contractor, clearly on the defensive. I made the young labourer sit up and offered him water. It seemed like a muscle injury, nothing that a few doses of anti-inflammatory and painkillers could not cure.

Over time, I learnt that the contractors were always on the defensive when their labourers got injured as they were liable for prosecution. For that reason, they were always courteous to me. A favourable report from me could save them thousands of rupees to ward off a police investigation.

Working at the stone crushers was a labour-intensive job, so no one could afford to employ sick workers. There were plenty of 'fresh off the boat from Bihar' faces available on the sidelines. Whenever a worker arrived at my clinic, he would say, "Please call me first as I have to get back to work."

The Rajokri workers always received a preferential number in the queue. I would give the full course of medicine to them so they didn't need to come again. Every trip to the clinic cost them much more in deducted wages. I hesitated to give treatment for more than a week, but the labourers insisted on taking the complete course of the medicines, as visiting my clinic was a cumbersome option for them. Soon, it became the trend in the clinic to give even a month's medicines if required. Since I was careful with the doses, it worked well for short and long-term treatments. No one had any side effects. I think I was plain lucky, or maybe I just took that little extra care in communication. They were encouraged to call up on the phone for any problems.

These labourers were not arrogant or judgemental like some of the Bijwasan folks. They were humble and agreed to take whatever treatment I prescribed for them. However, they did not take 'Rest Advised' on the prescription very seriously. A leave longer than three to four days would leave them jobless. It was a sad situation, but once I had learnt all the nuances of the situation, I was more empathetic towards the labourers. It was imperative that they got well as quickly as possible. I learnt the true meaning of poverty from these people. I witnessed their strength and resilience and lack of any resentment for the rich. At times, a labourer would come to the clinic, all bathed, shaved, hair oiled and shoes polished to perfection.

"I am going home today," said Sai ram, one of the gentlest men. He smiled and his teeth gleamed in his dark, sunburnt face. "Please give me some vitamins and health powder for my wife."

They wanted vitamins and protein powders for their wives. I found it very quaint.

"How many days do you want it for?" I had to ask.

"She is pregnant for four months so give me vitamins for

five months," he said happily in anticipation of a new arrival. The naivety of these men never failed to touch me. I knew that Sairam had been in Rajokri for over seven months and hadn't visited his village during this time. Who was I to deflate his buoyancy over petty paternity issues? I handed him the required doses. This was a common topic of discussion with my colleagues. We found it amusing that the wives, back in the village, would get pregnant even when their men were thousands of miles away in Delhi. India was steeped in ignorance and illiteracy. Better ignorance than ill will.

One of the men, Gottu, enlightened me. "Madam, in our village our wives get pregnant by the letters we send." When I looked bemused and unbelieving, he said earnestly, "It happens in my village, what would you know?" There was no way to talk him out of it. I learnt to leave certain beliefs alone and not meddle in their innocent convictions.

It was not long before I realised that the residents of Rajokri came to me mostly for a chronic cough and breathlessness. Working on the stone crushers clogged their lungs and wreaked havoc with their immune systems. It is a well-documented fact that silica is released in the air when stones are crushed. This can cause fibrosis and permanent scarring of the lungs and can manifest even a decade later. The damage to the lungs is irreversible and incurable and called *pneumokoniosis* in medical lingo. It was made worse by beedi smoking, which was common in both males and females in Rajokri.

I presumed that the cough and shortness of breath was caused by the dust from the stone crushers or beedi smoking and, of course, tuberculosis. As much as they tried to soothe their coughs by gargling and syrups, the coughs just would not go away and the fever would be recurrent and intractable. It was obviously tuberculosis which formed a passionate bond with the stone dust-fed lungs. In fact, tuberculosis became so rampant in the nineties that any patient from Rajokri was a tuberculosis suspect.

Anorexia and weight loss were the first symptoms, but as they were working so hard at the quarries, with minimal food, they never noticed the loss of a few kilos. I did not have much awareness about tuberculosis and had never really seen a tuberculosis patient during my residency in Lady Hardinge. There was a different ward for these patients and we never went there. Tuberculosis seemed irrelevant back in the early eighties, so no one gave much attention to it. However, I excelled at diagnosing and deciphering X-rays, thanks to the countless hours spent in the Radiology Department, and I could pick out the slightest and earliest indications of this deadly disease. A patient could walk in, get X-rayed, diagnosed and prescribed treatment, all within an hour. Initially, I was the 'Jack of all trades' as I had no radiographer to take and develop the films. Loading the film into the cassette, clicking it, unloading it from the cassette, putting it in the developer and then the fixer, hanging it to dry and then reporting it was a tedious process. Shuttling between the regular patients and the X-ray patients became unsustainable. I designated an hour for radiology. Later, I found a good radiographer.

I read all the studies I could find on tuberculosis and gathered information from colleagues in the Infectious Diseases Centre in Delhi. I stocked the clinic with all the medicines that were needed to follow the latest regimen. In the eighties and nineties, I diagnosed about ten to fifteen tuberculosis patients a day. The moment a patient started to cough blood, the quacks would quickly wash their hands off them, which is when they came to me. The majority of patients coughed up lots of blood, and the sight of the crimson liquid caused panic. After an initial X-ray and a weight and blood test to gain a baseline reference, I started the anti-tuberculosis treatment without much delay.

I explained the plan and the duration of the treatment to the patient, and they were out of the clinic and back to work in less than thirty minutes. Most of the patients preferred to take a full month's treatment, and I stressed on the intake of protein and vegetables as their diets were rich in carbohydrates and oils anyway. Two eggs, two cups of milk, two handfuls of peanuts for weight gain and two bananas. I knew from experience that a good diet ensured quick recovery from this disease.

Most of these patients were also addicted to tobacco, alcohol and paan masala and it was impossible trying to wean them off these substances.

I did not force anyone to stop their addictions completely as that was an unrealistic request. As a result, I followed my rule of two: I allowed them two cigarettes a day and two drinks in a week. After a while, this strategy worked for some patients. Consequently, they were also able to save money, which could then go towards more fruits and eggs.

As a GP, it's very easy to monitor recovery in a tuberculosis patient; one just has to pay attention. The appetite returns, the fever abates, and the cough flattens out in two to three months. Furthermore, the blood in the sputum reduces in two months. All patients feared blood in the sputum more than any of the other symptoms, so a clean sputum gave them reason to continue the treatment.

Some patients discontinued the treatment at this stage because they thought they had recovered, but this is when my acquired talent in communication came in good use. Incessant phone calls urging them to come to the clinic, the lure of incentives, fear of a relapse, offering discounts, and any other tactics that would bring them back—I tried them all without any qualms; as a result most of them returned without a fuss.

"If you don't complete the treatment," I would say, "you will spread it to your family." Fear of causing a fatal spread within the family worked.

The government had introduced the DOTS (Directly Observed Therapy) scheme where the patients were called into the primary health centres twice a week to take the medicines. Principally, it was a well-meant scheme because the earlier one where they were given a monthly treatment to be taken at home was a failure. Both schemes used effective medicines, but they failed and the tuberculosis cases in the country rose each day. The fault lay in the lack of communication. The nurses and clinicians behaved as if they were handing out dole money. Self-respect is highly important to the poorest of all. Patients, who had received bags containing free, perfectly good medicines from the dispensaries, would dump these into the bins with the hope of a fresh start. The government DOTS program was not a success as expected due to many reasons.

Firstly, the patients received incomplete medications most of the time. Out of the four drug regimens which were advised for the first two months, the government supplies were never enough—patients only received two or three drugs at a time. On the second visit, patients would get the other two which were missing in the first month, leading to resistance and relapse. The primary healthcare centres would rarely be manned by doctors. Apathetic and uninformed paramedics would hand the patients whatever was available, so the poor patients returned home with just half the drugs and no instructions. Many patients who had religiously taken the DOTS for six months would still cough up blood and their X-rays displayed massive consolidation in the lungs with no improvement at all.

Secondly, the conviction of the patients for the treatment was zero. The paramedics could not explain and did not care enough to convince the patients that the treatment was important. No one realised that tuberculosis was not a medical problem alone but also a socio-medical entity. The DOTS treatment was used as a whip, but all that the patients needed was compassion and empathy.

Thirdly, DOTS was only prescribed for six months, which was not enough. The bi-monthly X-rays I did regularly proved that patients needed the treatment for a full nine months to ensure complete recovery.

When patients visited me with blood in their sputum even after taking DOTS for six months, I was confused at first. I wondered if their lack of recovery was due to MDR (Multi Drug Resistance), and I even worried whether I had missed a malignancy. For those who don't know, MDR raised its evil head in the late nineties along with HIV. The newspapers carried reports telling us how fatal MDR could be for most people and how treatment was very expensive. I set up a plan to try and treat these patients with regular tuberculosis medicines. I gave them four weight-optimised doses for three months and three drugs for another six months. Because MDR preyed on my mind, I was prepared to refer the patients to a chest hospital. From 1995 to 2020, I had only referred one patient who I thought had MDR.

As the world battled with MDR tuberculosis, I had almost a hundred percent success rate. If a patient missed a few days of treatment, my staff called them up relentlessly until they showed up at the clinic. I believe that MDR happened as a result of careless treatment.

The patients who left their treatment midway were partially to blame, but the responsibility largely lay with the person who administered the drugs. When I started any patient on an anti-tubercular regimen, it was a half-hour drill to explain the importance of the complete treatment. I threatened them with no entry to my clinic, and whatever else I could think of, if they left the treatment midway.

The taboo and hesitancy involved in accepting tuberculosis as just another disease also allowed it to spread throughout the community, so it had to be dealt with sensitively. The moment I announced that someone's husband had TB, their faces fell and they hurled a tirade of accusations my way.

"Your machine is faulty."

"You don't know anything."

"You are lying."

So I gave TB another name: pneumonia, which they accepted well. I did not see anything wrong with this small lie as long as they took the treatment. However, for women it was worse. Many husbands threw their wives out of their homes the day they were diagnosed with tuberculosis. The wives would be packed off to their parents' home. Some women who were not thrown out were treated like outcasts. If someone else in the household caught a cold, the woman would be blamed. In the early 2000s, I diagnosed a young mother with tuberculosis. She was not an open case and did not need to be isolated as there was just a slight haziness in her lungs. However, one day she came to me distraught, with tears flooding her face. I looked at her and she said, "My husband fell off his bike and hurt himself."

"So?" I asked.

"My mother-in-law beat me up," she replied sobbing. "She blames me for bringing misfortune to the family."

Her situation was extremely unfair, so I decided to stop calling tuberculosis by its tainted name. If it were an open case, I would just inform her relatives that she needed to rest and should stay away from other people to build up her strength. My plan worked and saved many women from homelessness and untreated tuberculosis. Ironically, the majority of the patients with tuberculosis were men and the women were catching it from their men.

As the years went by and the internet became more accessible and popular, patients could google the names of the medicines I prescribed and they would march up to my clinic angry and betrayed. "You didn't tell us you were giving TB medicines!" they would exclaim as they flung the medicines at me.

This turn of events bothered me, so I had to change my strategy again. The patients had to be told the truth. A lot of explaining and counselling was needed. It was ironic that all the patients who discontinued the treatment were the educated ones and had access to the internet.

Children were also not spared by this disease. They came with lack of appetite, loss of weight, pain in the abdomen, and a mixture of loose stools and constipation, which were all helpful in reaching the diagnosis. Most of the time the symptoms were ignored as rarely did they display lung involvement. An ultrasound of most of these children showed abdominal lymph nodes which clinched the diagnosis of tuberculosis. After diagnosis began the hour-long argument of trying to convince the patient's parents of it. Although most of them agreed, some walked away in disbelief. These kids improved incredibly fast.

Believe it or not, a GP has to be well-versed in prices of common food items. Most of my colleagues made the mistake of prescribing unrealistic treatments and food, but I delved deeply to find the affordability factor for anything I prescribed. To hand over prohibitively expensive protein powders and vitamins was counterproductive, because if a patient could not afford treatment, they were more likely to discontinue after a month or two. I also took their daily earnings into account and then devised a meal plan for them.

As more and more tuberculosis patients required funding, I wish I had cultivated some people who had a clout in the political circles. Maybe I should have told my stories at the parties I attended. Perhaps the wine clubs where rich burgundies flowed, and the rotary clubs that sponsored lavish dinners in five star hotels would have funded a few patients. But I doubt something useful would have come out of those parties. I know how easy it is to click one's tongue and look appropriately sad. Very few remember the commitments made while sipping wine.

It saddens me even today that many TB patients had to be turned away without medication due to lack of funds. In the nineties, a labourer did not earn much, yet most agreed to take the treatment as being bedridden was not an option for them.

Once a family that consisted of the husband, his wife and

sister all had tuberculosis in various stages. They came to me from Shahbad. This small hamlet was an hour away by bicycle.

"Let me get myself treated first," the man said naively. "Then you can treat my wife, then my sister." His plan sounded plausible, but I knew it wouldn't work. The piecemeal approach would never eradicate this disease from his family.

Somewhere in the late nineties, HIV also crept into the picture. The diagnostic lines between tuberculosis and HIV were indistinguishable and indistinct.

CHAPTER NINETEEN

Then Came Maggi Noodles and More

IN THE EXCITING nineties India was overwhelmed and corrupted with the decadence of new goodies from the west. I sensed that something hugely different was happening in India. I experienced globalisation first-hand from the people who were affected by it. The flurry of globalisation hit the country like a deluge and it spared no one.

It started in 1991 when the import duties were reduced and foreign investments flooded the country.

I didn't need to read about the Indian economy touching 3.5 billion of imports or about the relaxation of import duties in the newspapers. When every single shop in every village was stocked with foreign chocolates, cheese and chewing gum, it was difficult to be unaffected by the euphoria that engulfed every single person. Local grocery stores displayed a profusion of glossy bags of Hershey's, Toblerone, cheese slices, mustard sauce, Tabasco, sandwich spreads, relishes and many kinds of pasta and breakfast cereals. The inflow of all these imported things in a country that was starved of quality goods since the independence, was bound to cause tsunamis. The retailers were laughing all the way to the bank.

I observed the enhancement of life due to the duty-free imports, even though it was more of a euphoria than an enhancement. A year later I was witness to the blight that followed—a blight that struck society in a permanent way. There were reports about the rising GDP of India but there were no reports about globalisation and its impact on health parameters, psychological issues, social disturbances and cultural costs. There are bars and graphs to measure economic data but there is no gauge to measure happiness of families, hopes and hopelessness, dreams and failures, and desperation of people.

Amartya Sen, the Nobel prize winner said, "GDP is a narrower measure of human development."

The collateral damage of progress caused havoc in large chunks of society and it went unnoticed. I experienced the hysteria and imbalance that the duty-free consumerism caused in urban and rural populations.

I learnt about the effects of these western goods not from journals or newspapers, but from people who lived in small houses that had no windows and no drains, yet spent a chunk of their pay on Maggi noodles.

From people who spent a large portion of their salaries to rent new movies.

From children of affluent families who could afford the best foods yet were malnourished due to their addiction to fast foods.

From substance-abuse cases that wreaked havoc in relationships and families.

From perfectly normal marriages that became disrupted.

And from the increased rate of suicides of young adults who didn't know what hit them.

I studied thousands of families in the new environment. A mother who came crying to me. "Please help me," she sobbed. "My son has started taking drugs."

Wives would walk in, "My husband hanged himself from the ceiling." People seemed to be losing their equanimity and sanity.

Some women would walk in bleeding from their face defaced by bruises, "My husband has become so violent."

One may wonder what did all these have to do with globalisation? It was a full circle. When the greed to acquire reaches such levels that all good sense and values are pushed away, then descends a darkness of unreason.

1991 saw the first satellite TV channel flash on the TV screens in every home. The educated were aware and informed but the illiterate labourers and villagers were caught off guard. Uncensored movies affected the simple minds of these illiterate people. The young emulated the movies in mind and body. They did not have the wisdom to discern the real from the make-believe.

Denim jeans, tight shirts and pop music filled the senses. The restless young minds adapted to the duality of identity. The western culture attracted them like a vice while the family roots held them back. There had to be a debilitating dissonance. All this was catalysed by the thousands of call centres that trained them in the right American accents. With the new accents, new movies and new clothes came the desire to live the new American dream. The girls thought it was an acceptable way of life to live in relationships. They would come to me confused when they got pregnant.

Of all the goodies that crept in insidiously, it was the breakfast cereals and Maggi noodles that changed the lives of women in India. Every woman was burdened with the morning chore of making fresh dough and rolling out fresh parathas with at least one vegetable curry for most meals. These processes were very elaborate and time-consuming and some breakfasts needed preparation the night before. These women had to wake up in the wee hours of the morning to wash, cut and cook the vegetables for breakfast. Along with that, they would start preparation for the mid-day tiffins. Close on the heels of that would be some lunch for the children as they returned from school. Evenings saw the women toiling away in the kitchens preparing dinner. The Indian meals, besides being labour-intensive, were divisive. Meals became important topics of discussion in the offices. The number of dishes in the tiffin, the quality of packing and the quality of the tiffin itself, were all indicative of a person's personal lifestyle and status.

Maggi brought uniformity to everyone's lives.

Instant noodles were the gift of the century. These noodles were made by many brands but it was the sheer strength of marketing that all instant noodles were known as Maggi. The entire family could sit at the table together to eat for the first time as one could get dinner on the table in two minutes.

One could keep up with the neighbours with a slight change in eating habits without derailing the budget of the house. However, the most prized and devoured item of all were Maggi noodles which only took two minutes to cook! What could anybody make in two minutes? There were two-minute commercials on TV showing happy moms and happier children gulping down spoonfuls in giant bowls. It was like mass seduction. Mothers felt they were being the quintessential, loving parent as they opened packets of those wiry things for their little ones. By adding a few vegetables, one could reduce the guilt of zero nutrients.

The wonderful Maggi noodles replaced milk, legumes, eggs, yoghurt, fruit—essentially everything. Maggi was the placating choice for a tantrum-throwing kid, coercing a kid to finish her homework, or blackmailing a kid to attend school.

New-age breakfasts offered a plethora of maple syrup and Oreo cookies, cheese slices and seasonings to choose from. Who wanted the stodgy and monotonous glass of hot milk, poha, dosas or parathas? The children would brag in the school buses about the new flavours of the cereal and Maggi in their tiffins. It was imperative to carry noodles and pasta in their tiffin or face ridicule from peers. I know of some children who would choose to sit alone in a corner to eat lunch, as other children would laugh and make fun of anyone who carried a mediocre-looking plastic tiffin which contained a paratha and vegetable. Parents had to fall in line even if they knew these were unhealthy choices. Packing cheese pasta into the kid's tiffin was a status symbol. This was the case with upper-class kids too.

Most importantly, these fast foods brought about a sense of amelioration in people's unremarkable lives. Westernisation brought with it advertisements that showed golden-haired, pretty girls having cold milk with cereal. All one had to do was to pour cold milk from the fridge and one was transported into the modern world.

Those who had travelled to the glorious land of the USA were familiar with these brands. All these goodies were now available without duty and in Indian rupees.

Then there were those who had never set foot in the magical duty-free shops at the airports, but had just heard stories from people who had. They had heard how cheese could be bought in slices and cubes and had heard of Uncle Chips in all its glorious flavours. They could now stand in a shop and select from endless choices.

Being a general physician, I watched the evolving food patterns of the urban, semi-urban and rural communities with a heavy heart. I was dismayed at what was happening but a doctor is not a policymaker.

Within a short time, the body weight of the kids declined and their immunity levels decreased. Lower immunity levels meant more kids came with respiratory infections. Lack of vitamins and protein intake had to take its toll, for there is no fast food that offers adequate protein and vitamins! The children had large abdomens and skinny limbs due to the carbohydrate-rich diet that lacked proteins. Their bloated abdomens signalled the onset of Kwashiorkor, a syndrome generally seen in poorer children with severe protein deficiency, but these youngsters were from wealthier households. Most of them were leading a passive life full of Maggi noodles and television. They looked sluggish, pale and dull, and their haemoglobin levels were even lower than 6 gms at times. Malnutrition, Kwashiorkor, anaemia and fatty liver cast their vile haze on children who were healthy a few years earlier. Interestingly, most of the incoming paediatric patients were boys.

It took less than four to five years for an observable and

recordable decay to set in. Mothers and teachers were clueless but I knew exactly what was happening.

I attempted to interpret the family dynamics to unravel this scenario and it became an interesting and compelling study for me. I spoke with each mother and grandmother about their cooking habits, and I asked about the tiffins the kids took to school. I knew where the problem lay but I was taken aback as I learnt the proportions of the problem.

It may seem trivial to some, but the excessive dietary shift in homes in India was alarming. The literate gave in to the temptation of quick and tasty fast food knowingly. It was the illiterate who bore the brunt of this new fad.

I do not think any research was done on this aspect. There was a WHO study around 2005 that stated that the weight of boys in India had reduced, along with other health criteria. No one could find a reason. I think I hit the jackpot when I discovered the reason for malnutrition in boys. Before the entrance of Maggi, the males of the family got the premium food cooked at home while the girls had the leftovers. I observed that the girls looked emaciated and had stunted growth, while their brothers glowed with health. The pronounced discrepancy in the health parameters disturbed me immensely. No amount of counselling and teaching diverted any extra food to the daughters.

After the advent of Maggi I saw these girls were getting the green vegetables, milk and eggs that were discarded by their brothers. As the novelty of Maggi wore off, people realised that the food costs were building up. Only the boys had the privilege to buy Maggi; the rest of the family was having the regular food. The little girls desired Maggi, but soon accepted that only their brothers could have them.

"What does he eat?"

"Oh, he eats a lot," the proud mother would echo.

"How much money do you give him to spend daily?"

Enthusiastically, the mother would say, "He takes about fifty or sixty rupees daily. He loves to eat outside food. There is so much fruit and milk lying at home but he doesn't have those so I have to give it to my daughter instead."

"Does she also eat outside food?" I would ask.

"No, no," came a defensive response, "she doesn't want all that stuff; she likes her vegetables and dals."

Even though the food at home was good for the girls' physical health, they continued to crave those goodies too because they felt left out at this overt discrimination.

The boys then became hooked to the fad of the 2000s—momos and chow mein! Decades afterwards, in rural areas, it is still the boys who get to eat all these and show signs of malnutrition and stunted growth. The girls get to eat home cooked food and glow with good health.

"Don't you want to become like Akshay Kumar, tall and handsome?" The favourite movie star tactic worked at times with the boys.

When too many parents started to come, distraught, I proposed the approach of smart eating. My talks in various schools started with, "Yes, you can have Maggi noodles, burgers and ice creams but smart eating is the solution."

My formula involved two cooked meals at home, two pieces of fruit, two eggs, two tomatoes and two glasses of milk every day. Every Sunday, they could have two kinds of junk food. Their simple minds accepted this simple formula of 'two' and adopted it. I present this formula to all pregnant women and developing adolescents also. My rule of 'two' has always functioned better than giving them long food lists.

The gender bias could be seen at many levels. The boys were sent to private schools while the girls were sent to the free government schools.

This bias too bounced, like the Maggi fiasco, as the government schools had more stringent rules and better teaching. The girls performed better in the final certificate examinations whilst the boys floundered, barely scraping though. So deep were the gender biases, they were heartrending. I saw that the boys had shoes, socks and a sweater in winter, while their little sisters were in their cotton frocks, shivering barefoot in my clinic.

"Where is her sweater, where are her socks and shoes?" I would ask.

"She doesn't wear a sweater, she doesn't like to," the mother would answer quite unperturbed.

CHAPTER TWENTY

Early 2000s and Sackfuls of Money

"All things truly wicked start from innocence."
Ernest Hemingway

DURING 2002 AND 2003, farmland prices increased to dizzying heights after a ten-year slump. It happened without warning and caught everyone off guard. My brothers sold the eight acres of Father's farmland just as the prices began to rise; they assumed it was a good time to do so. Little did they know that prices would quadruple in a few months. After my brothers sold the land, I was left without the comfort, security and pride I had of the land that Father had bought. The prices continued to rise. This was a gold rush by all standards. Everyone wanted a piece of the golden pie. The sleepy hamlets of Kapashera and Bijwasan became the most expensive pieces of real estate in and around Delhi. Suddenly all my friends who used to turn up their noses at Kapashera and say, "Where? In Delhi? Never heard of it!" were now in awe of my place of work.

"Oh, Kapashera, I have a friend who lives there; it's coming up really well." At least now I could say with pride that my clinic was in Kapashera. No more was I ashamed of the place. Kapashera became the buzzword of the decade.

An elevated work place status for me was the least of my worries at that time. I had to witness and deal with a new set of problems that this fresh money brought with it. They were new problems and I had to start learning again, casting aside the complacency that I had fallen into.

Most of the Bijwasan folks sold off their land and so did the Kapashera people. They sat on millions in their backrooms. In the natural series of consequences, some changes were good but a lot of them were extremely ugly. Urbanisation and unreasonable affluence gnawed at the social mores, ethics and morals. This change was worse than what had happened in the nineties when globalisation arrived on the scene.

A tremendous social upheaval was taking shape.

On close observation, I figured out the strange dynamics of this society. I discovered that it was the older men, the fathers and the grandfathers who owned the wealth. These old men sat on charpoys and smoked hookahs and played cards all day long. It was the clan's duty to keep filling the hookahs with tobacco and keep the old man in good spirits. The freshly-made food, cooked on new gas stoves, was handed to him by the veiled daughter-in-law. The father-in-law was the most pampered one in the family as he was the one who had the money and doled it out to each family member every single day. No one wrote a will so everyone fell over themselves to be in his good books.

"I will give my money to anyone who looks after me," was the popular criterion to distribute wealth.

On close interactions, I gathered that the people who had sold their land received payment in sackfuls, which were kept in small rooms at home. No one I knew in Kapashera trusted banks. The concept of investing hadn't taken root in the 2000s. They were farmers and land was the only option for them. So, what did they do with all this money?

It was obvious that the unused money that lay in the house gave rise to discontent amongst the younger males. They started to bully, torture and even abuse their father to force him to part with the money so they could live the life of their dreams. There were rumours of old men passing away in their sleep or suffering from sudden heart attacks at night. The real causes were uttered in hushed whispers in the back lanes—whispers of the old men being strangled, smothered or poisoned by their sons.

After the passing of the father, the eldest son held the reins of the wealth and would divide it amongst his brothers as he thought fit. The sisters, obviously, had no claim to any money.

What does one do with millions lying in huge sacks in small dingy rooms? I heard about these rooms from disgruntled family members. "He has two rooms full of money but he doesn't give me anything."

Well, they rebuilt their homes into lavish bungalows and bought the most expensive, most shiny sofas. They brought home the largest fridges, coolest ACs and, of course, their window into the world, the televisions. The TVs they bought were the most expensive and were large, really large. Families bought big, swanky cars, which were freely available now after globalisation. Gone were the farmer clothes; they bought boxes of Reebok and Nike trainers and sweatpants. Sports shoes and sweatpants became a uniform code for the young, and signified new money. The men looked dandyish, just like in the Bollywood movies.

The women had it good too. They got their hair done and painted their nails for the cattle were sold and there was no more cow dung to be collected, and no fodder to be cut every morning. Many beauty parlours sprang up overnight to cater to the frenzied demand.

As a result, life was good.

No more dung cakes, no more milking of the cows, no churning of the butter and no more blowing into the wood fires. Some of these changes were good for the women as I saw that with a decreased workload, they looked better and took more care of their children. Their children started to do better in school and pursued higher studies; some even went abroad to work.

The shoes, cars, beauty parlours and lavish homes did not even make a tiny dent in the sacks of the green bundles that lay around. So, what else did they do?

The Big Bang of the 2000s was much bigger than the liberalisation of the nineties. A new brand of shops opened as some of the young men did not like the idea of sitting idle. They opened showrooms of Reebok, Adidas and Nike. Some opened restaurants and gyms. The majority of them became real estate agents and builders because more people wanted to buy the leftover farms.

The farmlands that were being sold to rich people needed to be developed into fancy homes with lush bathrooms, beautiful interiors, swimming pools and tennis grounds. Some of the men opened ancillary units that provided farm accessories. Stone quarries that stocked the priciest Italian marble, tile shops for beautiful bathrooms, wood shops selling doors and windows—all these and many more mushroomed.

The more adventurous built multi-storied buildings on

some part of their farmlands. These buildings brought in bagfuls of rent adding to the bags already lying unused, yet it was better than squandering it away on alcohol, drugs and mistresses. Gradually, before I realised, rows and rows of shops lined the roads with swanky glass exteriors and those who built these homes and shops for rental are still reaping the benefits. Earlier, my clinic stood out as an urban structure, but amidst all these multi-storied constructions, it looked more rural than ever.

Several DVD shops opened so people could rent movies and watch them on their new televisions. The demand led to availability, following the simple economics principle of demand and supply. Almost everyone had a TV by then. It was obvious that the DVD shops flourished also because the internet and dish TV were not introduced in India at that time. Bollywood dominated the minds of this vulnerable population with its risqué songs. I continued to witness major social changes and society was changing so fast that I could barely keep pace. I could not imagine how my simple villages had changed so much. I missed my simple village folks. With all this money, people were no longer bound to the farm work for there were no farms. Work and a lifestyle that was theirs for eons was cast away like a diseased organ.

There's not much anyone can do with money after a certain point.

In about two years, I witnessed the ill-effects of all kinds of addictions. There was no choice; I had to because I was the first port of call for families who faced problems. Where else would they go?

Women who had been beaten, battered and thrown out, suicides, and attempted murder were the commonest to set foot in my clinic. When brought in by the family, I had to rely on my experience, gut feeling and intuition. No machines could diagnose whether the husband was lying that it was suicide or she had been poisoned; whether I could treat her in my clinic or whether she had to be referred to Safdarjung Hospital. The complexities of an FIR (a police report), had to be kept in mind although they were not very common those days. The family pleaded and begged for me to treat the abused victim in the clinic because no one wanted to go to Safdarjung and answer uncomfortable questions posed by relatives, the police and doctors. It was strange that all the victims happened to be women because it seems that a female is the punching bag in society. Drugs, alcohol, womanising, abuse and rapes were all in the male domain.

There were the more sinister cases of the burnt brides. Some were brought to me almost dead and the others were just cremated. I witnessed a sizeable number of burnt brides. They were always brought in too late. It was obvious that no one wanted them to be saved, as saving them would defeat the purpose of setting them on fire. This was the late 1980s when a bride was pushed into the flames after being doused with kerosene. She was brought lifeless and burnt within a few minutes of the incident. Her husband and mother-in-law accompanied her. As they lay her on the examination bench, I moved closer to the burnt victim. My stomach twisted with nausea and the smell of burning flesh seared my senses. I had never seen or smelt freshly-burnt flesh so close before. I could see that her shirt had fused with her skin and could not be pulled apart. The smoke still singed her skin. The flesh had started to gather into wrinkles and curdle as a paper would.

How can anyone forget such visions? Her eyes, still alive, looked at me beseechingly. She pointed with her gaze. Since her arms were scorched too, I could not spot them in the wrangled mass. As I went near her, I heard a soft stutter of a whisper and followed her gaze which moved around the room. It moved from her husband to her mother-in-law and stopped. "She threw kerosene on me and then a lighted match," gasped the burnt woman. I looked at the mother-in-law accusingly.

"She was cooking food and her dupatta caught fire," said the old woman. I looked at the husband with many unsaid questions. He looked back and knew that I knew. Men rarely inflict cruelty on women unless goaded by another. They could be blamed for being gutless and not standing up to their mothers. Spineless and effete! Yet being weak was not an absolution for the torture of their wives.

I shuddered at these happenings.

Single young women started to visit me complaining of stomach pain. Soon I discovered that stomach pain in a young woman meant that she was pregnant. After relentless history taking I carried out the mandatory urine test.

"You are pregnant," I would inform these young women.

"No Doctor, that's not possible," the denial was automatic and expected. "I am not that kind of girl." The denials would turn aggressive. "You know me, doctor, I used to come to you earlier with my mother; maybe your test is wrong." She would look at me accusingly. "You know I belong to a good family, I can't be pregnant."

They were right in saying that I knew them. They were not that type of girls. They were nice girls who had lost their way home. Most of them had visited my clinic since they were toddlers, but I was correct too—they were almost always pregnant. The girls were not to be blamed as they didn't know any better. It was a lifestyle affliction.

"You will have to come with your mother," I advised every girl under eighteen. The mother had to be involved to continue further action.

There was no way I would break rules after incessant tutoring by my husband. The mother had to be involved to continue further action. The next day the girl would come to the clinic with her mother. It was heart-breaking to break the news to the mother knowing that she would wail loudly, start beating her chest and her daughter, or worse of all, call up her husband. No matter how gently I broke the news, every mother exploded. Very often they blamed me for giving wrong information and keeping bad-quality testing kits. This was the denial phase.

"You must be wrong, your test must be wrong!" most mothers would exclaim. "My daughter is not like that. There has to be a mistake. Her father will kill her."

After their initial outburst, some sort of acceptance would creep in. I would advise the mother, "Keep this to yourself," to avoid any harsh reactions from the other people in the family. Some agreed, but others did not. I explained gently that their daughters were not to be blamed.

"Maybe the boy pestered her and she got carried away." These strategies worked and I got better at convincing them so the girls were not harmed or killed.

"Will her husband be able to make out?"

"No, never," I would assure them.

Parents who were more reasonable agreed for their daughters

to have the Menstrual Regulation, a procedure I had trained in. I assured them of its simplicity, and it took just a couple of minutes. The patient could return home within half an hour. However, I could do this procedure only for early pregnancies, and it was often too late for some.

If I had to name a single procedure that saved hundreds of lives and families, it was Menstrual Regulation. It was a simple, inexpensive, safe and unobtrusive procedure that allowed hundreds of girls to shake off the stigma of being an unwed mother. Many of these girls are now happily married. Sad is a situation where a girl has to bear the burden of a moment's weakness all her life.

To my chagrin, pregnant schoolgirls as young as twelve started to visit me! The pregnancies were mostly due to mutual consent. It was easy to make out that the girls were precocious as they sported bikini wax from the various neighbourhood parlours. I don't know what was worse—the underage pregnancies or a bikini wax on a minor! Along with the pregnancies, they would visit me with all kinds of infections in all kinds of places where they shouldn't ever be. Just the coy look in the girl's eyes and the 'come hither' way they walked was enough for me to guess the problem.

Once I started doing early abortions, I saw the women grow more confident and liberated for now they had things under control. I introduced them to IUCD (intra-uterine contraceptive device) and oral contraceptives. Initially, most women were suspicious and sceptical of them, but after a lot of convincing they agreed. Eventually, it became a viable and acceptable option for women. When other women saw that these women looked better (due to fewer kids) and did not need monthly abortions, they all wanted their own IUCDs. The oral contraceptives also became socially accepted.

As wealth permeated into the yarn of the society, the ill effects and rot became apparent. One of the wives came to me one day in a flood of tears. She had visited me with her husband and children a couple of times in the past.

"He is drunk all day, every day," Rewati burst out.

"But your husband looks so sensible and grounded," I replied, surprised by her husband's transformation.

"I know, but ever since his father died, he has so much money and is always surrounded by friends," she sobbed into her dupatta. She continued to sob silently and said, "He got drunk yesterday evening and threw a pile of dollars into the air."

"Dollars?" I exclaimed.

These were new heights or rather lows, I thought to myself.

"Yes, he bought a lot of one hundred dollar bills to reduce the volume of the sacks," she added so I could understand. "After a few drinks he took the dollars and threw them in the air." I pictured the green bills being hurled into the air, wafting a bit, before falling to the ground. Little did people know what hellish devastation these riches caused in thousands of lives. I learnt that coming into money was not a pleasant occurrence, contrary to what everyone believed.

Meena was one of the prettiest women I had seen in real life. She was doe-eyed, tall and slim, with a disarming smile and a glowing complexion. She would come smiling on some days and eyes filled with tears on other days. She would come at times with, "Look doctor, I have gained so much weight," or "I have this pigmentation on my face." She was aware of her beauty and I would just smile and advise her. The first two years of her marriage had been blissful and she would be like a ray of sunshine each time she walked into my clinic.

Then the inevitable happened!

Her husband sold off a part of their farmland. That meant a cool few lakhs of new money. He acquired new friends, new gangs, and new respect from freeloaders. A happy family was driven apart. Physical violence, abuse and alcoholism took its toll. Once Meena came and her face was covered with her dupatta.

"What happened to your face?" I asked instinctively as I had never seen her face covered. I knew the answer even before she could say something.

"He slashed my face with a knife," she said quietly. Her eyes were dry. She had probably shed all the tears she had. I know there comes a time in everyone's life when one is left with no more tears. The eyes remain dry and the heart remains cold and free from emotions. Meena had a stony look about her.

"Why?" I could muster no other word. "Why did he do that?"

"He said that he will spoil my pretty face so no one will look at me." She started to sob into her dupatta.

"Call him in."

"No, he won't come in, he is standing outside. He is embarrassed to face you," she explained. After much coaxing, he came in. "My friends…it was my friends who challenged me to beat her up," he said, clearly apologetic. "They said…if I were a man I would beat up my wife."

I cleaned up her wound. "I will stitch it up nicely," was all I could offer. "Why don't you lodge a police complaint?" I said as indignation set in.

She seemed to agree as I could see a ray of comprehension settle on her pretty face.

"The bashing is increasing by the day," she moaned. "He threw a flower pot at me just a week ago."

She sat for some time in the clinic sobbing silently. I heard her calling up her father and brothers and narrating the story to them.

"My father is coming to get me." She smiled amidst her tears and waited in the clinic till her father came to fetch her. As I saw her receding back on the father's bike I hoped some solution would be found.

I didn't see Meena for a few months after that incident. Later I heard that she had got a restraining order from the court which banned her husband from coming within twenty meters of her. A few months later, she entered with a box of sweets in her hands. "This is for you," she smiled. "Please bless me; I have opened a tailoring shop."

"That's wonderful." I was truly happy for Meena.

She continues to visit me on her brand new scooter wearing her brand new helmet.

Sadly, the most common injuries were to the vagina! The women never revealed the correct history to protect their husbands or to protect their dignity. Extracting the cause of injury was like talking to silent walls. Invariably, the explanation they gave was, "I fell over a bucket." Sometimes it was the tap, other times it was a slip on the floor even when I knew these women concealed the real reason. I quietly stitched their cuts and did not pry into their unseen wounds. Professionally, I liked stitching the cuts and wounds as I dealt with them with an artist's finesse and was proud of my job. It filled me with joy to see the clean surfaces when they healed so beautifully. It is very important to study the economic dynamics of a society while working as a GP.

I talked to the men freely, sometimes sternly; at other times the role of a psychotherapist was thrust upon me and I savoured it.

Instead of chiding them for hitting their wives, the praise worked better. "You are educated; you are from a good family, so why do you drink so much?" This approach worked on some young men.

I remonstrated gently and firmly, never belittling them in any way.

In times when patients were getting to be aware of their own rights and the doctors were treated with so much mistrust, I banked on my reputation and communication skills to help me out.

Just before large amounts of new wealth corrupted everyone, education was held at a premium. It was considered prestigious to send a child to a good school. Every parent aspired to tutor their kid to their best ability. The parents would keep a close track on the child's grades and interact with the teachers on a regular basis. Private home tuitions were expensive but were arranged for most kids. I knew some patients would scrimp on their own clothes and shoes to pay for expensive tuition.

These values changed when DVDs and televisions came into the living rooms. The countless channels with movies and serials seduced the young and old alike. The parents and teachers were left overwhelmed with the sudden invasion of television in their homes. Watching unregulated and unlimited television, and playing computer games into the night seemed harmless initially but snowballed into an out-of-control situation very soon. Children started to visit me for headaches, irritation, loss of appetite and lack of concentration in school. Eighty percent of them failed their high school examinations. This percentage of failures soon increased to almost a hundred percent. They would glue themselves to the television sets as soon as they reached home. Throwing the school bags on the floor, they would grope for the remote control.

With sleepy eyes, groggy heads and guilty thoughts of schoolwork waiting to be finished, they would switch on the TVs. As if in a trance, they ate their meals and answered their mothers in monosyllables. When the teachers reprimanded the parents, the parents became distressed and stopped attending the PTAs.

Then they brought the wayward kids to my clinic for management because I seemed to be a solution for all their problems.

"Please give me some medicine for Golu, Doctor. His teacher says that he can't concentrate in class." Golu would sit across me, oblivious to the anxiety he was causing. Probably Golu was anxious to get back to the TV series he was hooked on.

There were no questions I could ask, and there was no diagnosis or treatment for Golu's affliction. I knew and the parents knew.

"Ok, just take these tonics, they will help him." I would hand over the tonics tiredly. "Try to stop the paid channels and get him off TV."

"Oh, but I like to watch some Hindi serials too; I can't stop the channels." The mother would become defensive.

The queue of these TV kids in my clinic became longer and

longer. The long hours the children spent watching television was causing a deficiency of sleep, food and exercise.

One of my staff girls hailed from Samalkha so she knew the reality. One day she blurted out, "It's been three years since any boy has cleared the board exams in Samalkha; everyone fails." I was aghast. The addiction to these enticements soon overtook good common sense in everyone, adults and children alike. After just a year or two, parents stopped bothering even if a child dropped out of school.

A bunch of teachers from the nearby public school were my patients, too, and dropped in for random consultations. A teacher once came into the clinic frustrated and angry saying, "What can one do if the parents don't mind?"

"The boys use such foul language," said a female teacher.

"I don't want to reprimand any of them; they carry knives to school," said another.

"Let them go to hell. We should just do our job and go home."

Even as the teachers turned a blind eye to the falling grades, the rowdiness and impudence of the children, especially the teenagers, made it incredibly difficult for them to control the students in the classroom. When they could not take the verbal abuse any longer, I noticed that they quit.

This was the same society that celebrated if a child in the village graduated from high school. The parents of these children were unapologetic and almost condoned their kid's behaviour.

"Oh, my son didn't like school," they would say casually.

"They learn nothing at school; colleges are worse," they claimed.

"Children get spoiled in college," some parents stated as they comforted themselves with this thought.

"It's okay if my son passes the sixth or seventh grade of school," the proud parents would lament. "After all, it's not as if he has to look for a job." Money was in plenty.

Since most parents weren't bothered if their children dropped out of school, marriage became the next step, especially for the daughters. The girls were married off at eighteen and the boys at twenty. The boys took care of their father's store until the ideal girl with enough dowry had been found for them from a neighbouring village.

CHAPTER TWENTY ONE

Boyfriend Season

DURING THE EARLY 2000s, I read about all the nice things that were happening to the youth of the country. The newly-erupted call centres were employing the youth in thousands. Large, white, air-conditioned taxis collected them from their homes and they were transported to work in air-conditioned offices. Their parents bragged about their children working in this environment and a general euphoria invaded the air.

Young girls looked and felt attractive in their new clothes. Dating and nights out with boys was inevitable. Intoxicated with youth, glamour and a new sense of financial freedom, the youngsters discovered the options and possibilities of dating and then there was no turning back. It was dangerous and exciting. Job environment, money and new clothes, mixed with recklessness of youth made an intoxicating cocktail. There was no place or patience for reasoning or sanity. When young people work together, both good and bad things happen. The young girls had boyfriends. Boyfriends meant mishaps.

I had a taste of this decadence in society, too. One of these cases which wasn't very pleasant had a long-term effect on my mental equanimity. This incident changed the way I looked at my patients.

It was a July afternoon around 1 pm.

I was packing to leave as I had to pick up my children from the school bus stop at two pm sharp. A well-dressed young lad came into the clinic.

"Can you please have a look at my wife?" I looked at him and ushered him in.

"What happened?" I asked, hoping that it was a small issue and I could leave for home.

"We were just going to Gurgaon to visit a relative when she started her periods and is bleeding a lot," he said in all seriousness.

I saw the girl walk in. She was wearing expensive clothes and I guessed they didn't belong to this rural area. I presumed they were newly-married as she was wearing the elaborate red bangles of a newly-married girl. As is my protocol, I sent the guy outside and took the history from the girl herself, thus precluding any harassment or duress.

"We got married two months back," she said a bit shyly. "I just started my period and it's more than usual." There was no reason to doubt her history. I had given her ample opportunity to let me know if there was any problem with her companion.

The two minutes that it took me for the history, I saw that my entire couch was soaked in blood. She was bleeding profusely.

I quickly called the husband from the outside room and told him, "I don't think she is too well, please take her to Safdarjung."

He pleaded, "Please do something, give her an IV at least."

This was more than twenty years back when I was still the idealist doctor. I didn't have the heart to turn them away without helping. I reasoned, an IV saline would surely help in this blistering July heat and could do no harm. I decided to give a fast drip as she was looking pale and a bit weak.

Twenty minutes later, I sent them off to Safdarjung Hospital with a prescription that said 'A history of bleeding for one hour. Referred to Safdarjung for further management'.

Next morning at 9 am, I got a frantic call from my clinic. "Please don't come today, the police are waiting for you." I was perplexed as to why.

There was no way of knowing the reason for the presence of the police in the clinic. What could have happened?

It was a scary situation. I stayed at home that morning wondering what could have happened. As I picked up the day's newspaper, the bold headlines screamed at me.

'Girl found dead in a white SUV outside Safdarjung Hospital'. Instinctively, I knew that it was the patient from yesterday. On reading the article, I learnt that there were four other boys in the van and the girl was gang-raped. So that was the cause of the profuse bleeding. The boys had taken her to SFJ as I had instructed. When they saw her collapsing, they probably panicked and left her in the van outside the SFJ emergency and fled for their lives.

My prescription was found in the van beside her body!

Well, that explained the police outside my clinic. This incident taught me never to hand out prescriptions generously as I was wont to do, especially to serious, referral patients.

By the next day, the culprits were traced from the vehicle

number. They were young so they quickly admitted to their crime. This incident further sharpened my clinical sense and intuitive skills and made me increasingly cautious and less idealistic.

A new profession carved its way into society. Young college girls made this into a business venture. To spend a few hours with men and earn handsomely was not a bad idea. However, a lot of unwanted pregnancies took place. I mention the topic of unwanted pregnancies yet again. By the end of 2000s, the magic MTP (Medical Termination of Pregnancy) pill stormed into the market, which was a godsend.

Besides unwanted pregnancies, I heard about abductions, suicides and murders. The fallout of liberalisation was dating and live-in relationships. Any girl who dared to befriend a boy from outside of her community was sure to meet a bloody end.

Unrequited love and doomed friendships were a tragic turn.

The one case I remember distinctly involved a pretty young girl who was brought to my clinic by her father. She was not eating anything; she stayed in her room and didn't talk to anyone. To get to the bottom of her loss of appetite, I sent her father out of the room so I could ask her some questions in private.

"What happened?"

"Is someone troubling you?"

"Any pain anywhere?"

But the girl sat in silence and stared at the ceiling.

Just when I thought there was no point in probing anymore, she spoke. "My boyfriend has found another girl," she revealed. "I do not want to live. If I stop eating then I will die." Her blank tone and expressionless eyes were screaming that she was struggling with depression. I called her father back into the room and expressed my fears. I sensed an imminent danger. "You need to look after her, don't leave her alone at any time," I warned her father. He did not pay heed to my words and laughed them off.

"My daughter is more sensible than she appears," he said.

"She can harm herself, please be careful," I repeated in a serious tone.

"She is a very sensible girl. I know my daughter, doctor," he said curtly and left.

I never heard from them again for another year. One summer afternoon, the same father walked into my clinic with slow, faltering steps. He was a shadow of his old confident self yet I recognised him immediately.

"Haven't you come before?" I asked, even though sure.

"Yes, I came with my daughter." He sat on the stool beside me. His face was devoid of the earlier hint of arrogance, I remembered. It had a pall of gloom and his eyes looked sad and defeated.

"You were right, Doctor. I was just passing by and saw the clinic was open, so I came in to say thank you," the father began. "My daughter..." he hesitated, "do you remember?"

"Of course, how could I forget her?"

The man sighed. "Well, she drank acid the very next week after we came to you...the entire gut got burnt."

I looked on with dread and misgivings.

"We got her admitted...a lot of operations were done on her in the last year. She has come home but is still bedridden." He spoke in broken sentences as he struggled to hold back his tears. My heart felt leaden with intense sadness and a lump formed in my throat. I needed to comfort him.

"It is God's will that she is alive. I am sure she will be ok after all the treatment," I muttered. It was inevitable that I changed as a person with every story that found its way in my clinic. How could I retain my intrinsic joy when I was living so many sad lives?

CHAPTER TWENTY TWO

Boys will be Boys

WITH QUICK ACCESS to wealth came a sense of entitlement in the youth. Rapes and suicides became the norm. Some took to alcohol, drugs and sex as this was something that money could buy very easily. The younger males wandered into new avenues and found exciting things to do. They learnt that they could go on fancy holidays with or without their wives, and that they could visit and stay in very posh hotels. They learnt that money was everything and the power it had on everyone. They sought new mistresses. This trend found its way into my clinic when men who earlier came with their wives started to bring their pregnant mistresses. "She is pregnant, doctor, please help me." It was amusing to know that none of them wanted to end the marriage. The mistresses were always 'just flings'.

The young men owned the latest SUVs with tinted windows; they smoked the most expensive cigarettes and found solace in the best alcohol money could buy. They moved in wolfish packs of four or five. They huddled up in their cars, stocked with premium liquor and latest music stereos with latest songs. Their pockets bulging with wads of cash, they were unstoppable. They crawled in the cars, scanning the streets for young girls. Any girl who caught their fancy was pulled into the SUV and gang-raped till they were satiated. They drove around the city or towards nearby fields to violate the girls, and then later, simply dumped them somewhere in the tall grasses. Usually the culprits could be tracked as the villages were close and word spread very fast. Blood boiled and feelings of revenge clouded all sanity. They were all Jats and blood ran hot in their veins. Some brothers would go and hack the culprits mercilessly.

Most families chose to remain silent when such incidents happened to their daughters. After all, the family name was important. Some of the patriarchs were harsher—they would lock the girl in a room without food or water for days till they could hear her silence. It was a matter of a few days and the young teenage girl would starve to death. Through no fault of hers, she had to bear the cross. No one ever got reported or punished for this barbarism as the neighbours understood and empathised with the family. The girls were declared to have died of natural causes. Some of these girls tied a dupatta around their necks and hanged themselves, to everyone's relief. The little wretched girl would slip out of this world into another, so quietly that no one would talk. By 2010, this menace of hounding the girls had serious fallouts.

Women were terrified of walking on the roads.

Parents were terrified.

Brothers were terrified.

There was a sense of foreboding every time anyone's sister

or wife or even mother stepped outside the house. This rot reached even the urban areas. Even though we lived in the poshest area of Delhi, I was also fearful for my daughter. She grew up without being allowed to walk anywhere outside the home after dark.

The reasons to rape were many. If there was a land dispute (which were plenty), the only threat anyone could give was, "Just wait, I will rape your sister." This was sure to make the opponent withdraw. It became the most potent threat anyone could throw at someone. The sister or daughter became a pawn in the name of family honour. Threats of rape and throwing acid on the face became common to wrangle property deals in one's favour. These threats were not mere empty words for they were uttered by Jats, so they were real and carried weight. There were enough girls who lived with acid-scarred faces to prove the threats.

Secondly, the undue importance given to virginity in India and the linking of the family honour to female virginity was the sole reason that vindictive rapes took place. Raping the wife, sister or daughter to settle any loans, property feuds, land disputes, rental problems and inheritance issues was a good solution. It seemed better than murder, too, as murder invited strict penalties.

Thirdly, it was the mothers' attitude towards their sons that 'boys will be boys' which paved the way for raising selfish monsters. Many rapes were without reason. They were a leisurely activity of idle minds. The rapes continue even today and newspapers blare the headlines about three year olds being raped and killed brutally. People have become desensitised to the news as there are so many things happening every single day.

All questions and fingers are raised at the girl.

Why did she go out with a male friend?

Why did she step out of the house after sunset?

Why was she wearing jeans?

Why did she not cover herself properly?

Very few were caught and fewer were punished, so the boys became arrogant and unafraid of the law. They widened their net for want of better prey and dared to frequent the five-star luxury hotels. Mayhem occurred when these boys acquired guns. The advent of guns was a potent concoction. The boys ended up shooting at random over trivial issues and at times they shot bullets in the air just for fun. They would shoot at weddings and at any celebrations. One would hear of accidental deaths. The punishment was mild, so was never a deterrent. If a bartender did not oblige with a drink quick enough, he was shot. If a girl did not reciprocate their overtures, the boys would shoot her. Some of these incidents like the Jessica Lal case appeared in the press and became infamous.

These boys who were shooting people in bars, raping girls in moving cars, keeping mistresses and beating up their wives at night, were my patients. Yes, they were all my patients! They looked normal enough. My female staff would throw me a silent glance if they recognised any of those boys or their misdeeds, so I was on my guard.

"Do you drink?" I would ask.

"Oh, never," they would reply, a bit too quickly. Quickly enough for me to know the answer.

"He brushes his teeth with whiskey in the morning," my staff would say. When I looked confused, they told me that it was a common phrase in the village for anyone who starts drinking at dawn. The crime graph in Kapashera and Bijwasan rose like the country's GDP, for the men were idle and lived in a constant state of inebriation.

CHAPTER TWENTY THREE

The Second New Bride

I REMEMBER THIS lovely family from Dhulsiras, a small village that was about 10 kms away, who would visit me once in a while. When the children were young, the visits were more frequent. There were three brothers in their family.

The eldest was a teacher at a government school and had a wife and two children. He seemed to be the sanest of the three. He was extremely quiet and spoke in monosyllables when asked about any ailments. His face remained expressionless and his eyes never met mine, but I knew that it was a mark of respect as he always looked past me at the wall behind. He usually came for his wife's ailments. I don't remember if he ever came for his own problems. His wife was a tall, lanky lady with a no-fuss attitude. She never smiled and usually came with complaints of weakness and general lethargy.

"How are you today?" I would begin cheerfully trying to elicit a smile.

"I am not well, I am never well," she would reply grumpily.

I could never put her complaints in any of my regular slots. A few placebos of multivitamins and a bit of calcium would get her going. Placebos always worked for her.

The second brother owned a small convenience store in the village. He was married and had two daughters aged ten and twelve years. His family seemed to be the healthiest as he rarely visited. The third brother was the youngest and the most vocal of them all. He was not married and was pursuing a postgraduate course. He had an air of covert disdain for the other brothers and one could see he held himself above them. I hadn't seen them for a year or so. One day, the eldest brother, the school teacher, came. I peered to see if his wife had followed him but I could not see her.

Maybe he wanted some medicine for himself, I thought. Then I noticed that the second brother's wife was standing at the doorway of my room.

"Come in, Nirmala," I invited her in with warmth.

The elder brother looked at me hesitantly. He opened his mouth to say something then closed it again. "Yes, so what brings you here today?" I said to put him at ease.

He again opened his mouth, hesitated, looked at me and then at his brother's wife. Then he kept quiet again. I was on tenterhooks by now.

"Yes, what is the matter?" I asked Nirmala.

"My brother died in an accident," he said with a solemn expression.

"Oh gosh, I am terribly sorry," I offered.

"This is his wife. She has some problems. Can you see her?" He pointed at Nirmala. I cast a casual look at him and then at the woman. He looked like his usual benign self.

What a harmless looking man this one is, I thought to myself.

I sent him outside as I usually do when I want to ask delicate questions to women.

"What happened to your husband?" I asked.

"He took poison," she said in a voice devoid of any emotion, "six months back."

I was taken aback by the tone of her voice.

I waited for her to tell me about her problem, but she remained silent and would not volunteer any information.

"Any fever?"

"Any pain anywhere?"

"Appetite?"

"Tiredness?"

"Headache?"

However many questions I asked, Nirmala kept quiet without any response but shook her head which meant a no.

"When did you get your period?"

"I missed my period," she uttered with her head downcast.

"Let me check your blood, maybe it's due to low haemoglobin," I said, since pregnancy was not on the cards.

Even as I said this, I knew what the problem was.

"No, no," she interrupted me. "Please test my urine."

After all these years, I had learnt to keep a deadpan expression even if I was shaken inside because I knew that if I appeared disturbed, it would put the patient on the defensive. Even if a pregnancy had been caused by adultery or rape, I had to remain calm.

"Ok, let's do that," I agreed. Not unexpectedly, the test displayed two red lines of a positive pregnancy.

"How come?" I had to ask directly.

"After my husband died, he took over my expenses," she revealed as she pointed to the eldest brother outside the room.

"That's nice of him," I replied to prod her on.

"I sleep with my daughters in one room," she continued, and then she started to sob. "Every night, when everyone is asleep, he comes and knocks on my door." She hung her head in sorrow. Looking at this diminutive figure, it took me a while to comprehend what she was implying, but once it dawned on me, my stomach twisted with nausea.

"Why don't you refuse?" I exclaimed with evident disgust.

"I can't, my daughters are sleeping in the same room; they are teenagers," she whispered.

I bent my head towards her to catch her words.

"I have to be very quiet or they will get up," she continued. "He comes every day, and today he has brought me to you. Every two months, he takes me to see a new doctor. I have already had three abortions since my husband died."

I burned with anger for the poor woman.

"Why don't you tell his wife and the rest of the family?"

"They all know," she said with a sniffle. "It's acceptable, since he is paying for our food and the children's education; he has a right."

Certain moments in a person's life become permanent memories, and this was one of them. As I listened to this frail woman, I internalised her pain and it engraved into my being as a permanent etching. I can still picture her sitting on that stool speaking softly so no one could hear. I could envision her lying in bed night after night, dreading his footsteps near her door.

I did whatever had to be done. I even convinced her to get an IUCD for protection against future pregnancies. I prescribed and inserted the contraception free of charge.

That night, I went home and penned a few distressed words which sadden me to this day:

The Widow
Dark oil lit lamp
Shadowing the room in flaccid
Mourning
Creaking in pleasure when he was there
Now
Phlegm like, she lies alone
Mopping, cooking, sobbing
All tasks done.
Nightfall, and the strange one creeps in
Beside her,
Like a village drain, she lies
Her wounds agape, retching silently
Lest her teenage daughters hear her
Whimper
Why did they not douse her in kerosene?
Or stone her into a gutter?

She was the first but not the last because after this woman I came across many more widowed women who were handed over to the husband's brother or cousin. He could be single or married with children of his own. Delving deep into this practice, I understood the benefits and the obvious sadness of it.

The helpless widow would get a man for all her needs and to help with her children; to take her to the doctor, and to buy her new clothes. The women had no choice. If there was no brother, then even a cousin or uncle could offer to marry her. She was available to anyone who was willing to bear the burden of the children. If she was pretty, she could choose between a few and she was spared the indignity and the helplessness of wearing the white clothes of a widow all her life.

It may seem strange to anyone who has not experienced life in rural India. One must understand that family and society are a much bigger entity than an individual can ever be. All big decisions of life i.e. job, marriage, children, choice of clothes and even the size of one's home, are all dictated by society and family. If a woman should have a third child or not, the mother-in-law decides. What kind of contraception the couple ought to use, whether they can go for a short vacation or not and whether they can be in the same room during her periods or not—these decisions were never personal. Nothing was ever a personal decision.

"How can they decide?" said one mother-in-law self-righteously. "They are too young, they can't make such decisions."

The points in favour of this seemingly unfair deal were that once a man accepted the widow as his wife, she was allowed to dress up like a married woman in bright clothes. She was allowed to participate in all festivities and enjoy all festivals, wear bangles, shiny clothes and eat whatever she wanted to, which a regular widow would not be allowed. She was even allowed to laugh. In return, the supporting relative or the second husband would get matrimonial rights.

This custom was popular because it also prevented the widow from asking for her property rights in the husband's share because now she was married to the other brother. Even if some educated women understood the motives of this custom, there was very little they could do. As long as they were not thrown out of the house, got food and shelter and their children could go to school, they were happy.

Some of them even found happiness in these second relationships. I explored this social custom more and questioned women who came to me in this situation. As I listened to their answers, I found it fascinating. When I saw that so many widows walked happily into my clinic with their new husbands, I realised that some mores were not as bad as they initially seemed for it worked for some, as many of the men were kind and compassionate. I know the feminists would batter me for endorsing this practice, but I have seen widows who were not absorbed in this social custom living a life of poverty, wearing shabby clothes, with their children having to drop out of school for want of financial support. This ritual was called *churi pehnana* (to wear a bangle), which still exists. The widows had no option as no parent ever took a married daughter back as the parental home belonged to the brothers anyway. However, things have now changed. With new laws in place, the parents give their daughters their share in land, and support her and her children.

CHAPTER TWENTY FOUR

The Big Fat Indian Family

EVEN AFTER ALL these years, I remember the day this sad looking young girl walked into my clinic. She walked ahead of her mother who followed closely at her heels. A benign looking man followed the two women. I looked up to see the threesome standing near my table. "Yes, what is the problem?" I asked. The man was obviously not a patient. I presumed he had accompanied his wife and daughter.

The mother was quiet and her eyes darted across the clinic furtively to gauge the extent of her privacy. Satisfied with the visual perusal, she sat on the chair in front of my desk next to her daughter. I took in her small form, crumpled garb and the pregnant silence without a word. She looked to be a simple lady, draped in a modest saree. Her face looked stony and did not allow an iota of expression to escape it.

She gestured to her husband to move out into the waiting room. With two quiet, tight-lipped women in front of me, I was left to my own devices to figure out what could have happened.

The girl's silent look of acceptance as she stared at the floor, and the mother's guilt-tinged demeanour gave me an idea of the problem. They seemed to be in collusion in their misfortune. What made my inference difficult was that I spotted no anger, no guilt, and no reaction whatsoever. No rebuke, no justification, no blaming, not anything. The hopeful look that most patients wear as they enter the clinic was missing.

"My daughter," the woman stuttered, "she has missed her period."

"Is she married?"

"No, she is only seventeen."

The obvious thing that struck me was how old and sad this girl looked. I could not imagine how a child of seventeen could manage to look so sad. At that point I understood the difference between a sad look and an unhappy look. The unhappy look comes when an unfortunate event happens, while the sad look is deeper, and comes when one has made peace with the event and feels helpless, knowing that nothing can be done about it.

Anyone could see that she had witnessed the reality of life first-hand.

I noticed the colour of her clothes, the way she kept her arms by her sides and the way she looked down at her feet—all these transferred some of that desolation my way too. Her face flashes before my eyes even decades later.

"When was her last period?" I asked. I had almost clinched the diagnosis and waited to hear if I was correct.

"She's two weeks late," the mother replied expressionlessly. I was correct so far. I sighed with relief that she wasn't any deeper into the pregnancy. "What happened?" I asked in a low, sympathetic tone.

I glanced at the young girl as I waited for an answer. She cast a look sideways at her mother asking for her permission to tell me the events. The mother nodded and let out a few silent sobs.

"When I was sleeping on Diwali night, he got drunk," said the seventeen-year-old. There was another long silence.

"Yes, and then?" I prompted gently.

"He got drunk and came into my room," the girl continued with a shaky voice as if reliving that miserable Diwali night. She was almost whispering lest 'he' heard.

"Who got drunk?" I questioned, fearing the worst. The girl raised her sad eyes to look at her mother asking for permission again. The mother nodded silently.

"My father!" The girl's words scythed through the air like a sharp blow. The mother shuddered as if the reality hadn't sunk in yet. She turned her head away to sob some more.

No wonder he had stood so confidently. He stood emboldened, assured of his safety for he knew his identity was safe. The girl's words "my father", hung in suspension in the clinic and the air in the clinic was silent for a few moments after the revelation. Probably it was sobbing too. I was sad and angry. Strangely, I wasn't angry with the father, but the mother. The woman who was protecting her husband. Why wasn't she screaming and ranting?

Why was she so accepting? She should have been raging mad. I seethed as I heard the events of the gut-wrenching reality.

How come the females could not react?

Would they burst into tears when home?

Would he beat her mercilessly once home?

I wish that I had not seen so much behind their faces. I should have limited my gaze to diagnosing the illness. Searching for too much in faces and trying to seek stories beneath them is tiring—so tiring that one forgets to live one's own life!

My staff stood with mouths agape. All eyes were on this melancholic girl.

My heart cried at her sadness.

It took me a while to get my professional demeanour back in place. However, once I had composed myself, I started to explain that it should be easy enough to manage the situation. "Don't worry, I can manage. No one will know," I assured them in a soft tone.

After I performed the MR procedure, the girl and her mother returned home and I could imagine that everything must have gotten to normal. The man must've quietly slipped out somewhere for a stroll. The two women would enter home quietly, without a word, and go about their chores in silence with lowered heads. They would cook for him, wash his clothes and make his bed.

This was a blow that time could not heal; friends could not heal. It was a cross that had to be borne by the girl alone. All her life. Rape by the father could never be shared with anyone.

When people experience so much dreariness in their lives, their emotions get blunted and they stop reacting. Back in Kalawati I believed that they were incapable of finer emotions. How wrong I was! I realised that the underreaction to tragedy was their safeguard against a complete breakdown.

Many girls visited my clinic after the seventeen-year-old girl and her mother. I never learnt to take these in my stride. The horrific rapes by neighbours were deplorable and angered me. The ones inflicted by loved and respected family members were even more despicable and deserved no forgiveness. The girls were sometimes as young as three or four years old. I never saw any mother ever raise an alarm. Was it self- preservation on her part at the cost of her daughter?

The worst part of these crimes was that the culprit was never indicted and his identity was protected energetically by the family. The mother could not throw out her husband or name her sons, nephews and uncles. She could not shame them in public as family honour was at stake. The victim was a young child who had no courage to stand up and point fingers. The rapist almost always got away scot-free and it was the victim who saved him.

What an irony!

Thanks to the big fat Indian family!

The barbaric crimes against young girls occurred in various settings.

Another case that disturbed me for days involved a young girl who was brought into my clinic by her sister and the sister's husband. The sister and the husband sat in front of me while the girl kept standing. Her curious, child-like gaze wandered all around my clinic and then settled on me. This girl looked about twelve years old.

The sister told me that they belonged to the hilly regions of Himachal Pradesh. Well, that explained the wide eyes and fair complexion, I thought to myself.

The little girl of twelve had been brought from the village to help out the older sister who was pregnant. There was nothing strange in this as it was the norm for younger sisters to come over and live with the elder one for a few months, till the baby arrived. The little girl started to fiddle and play with the paperweights kept on my table. I offered her some sweets. She happily took some from my palm and immediately popped one into her mouth.

"She has indigestion and a lump in her abdomen," said the pregnant elder sister.

"She has been complaining of pain in the stomach," added the husband.

I asked the young girl to lie on my examination table, and sure enough, I felt the lump her sister had described.

"Has she started her period?" I queried.

"No, she hasn't," replied the sister.

A tumour was the only diagnosis I could think of but she was too young for a tumour.

The idea of her being pregnant continued to bother me but the fact that she hadn't started her periods confused me. I knew that it was a delicate situation and I had to be extremely careful. An ultrasound would clear the air and I would have a firm diagnosis to work on. It took an hour for them to get the ultrasound done and reach my clinic with the report.

As I read the report my heart sank, for my fears were correct.

I faltered a bit and took a deep breath. They had to be told the diagnosis. I looked at the pregnant sister and then at her husband. The husband looked away, avoiding my gaze.

At that moment I knew that it had to be him.

The ultrasound showed a foetus growing inside the young girl. It was a twenty-week old foetus, alive and healthy. I could see the heart and the limbs and the spine of the baby.

"Your sister is pregnant," I said softly. The sister was astounded, angry, incredulous, all at the same time.

"How is this possible?" she stammered.

"Meenu hasn't even started her periods." Her disbelief was valid. My knowledge of science told me that probably it was the first month and she was about to start when a wayward egg found its way, got fertilised and got implanted in her tiny uterus.

The sister's face contorted in anger. She stood up and shouted, "You are a fraud. Your ultrasound is wrong; there is no one in the house except me and my husband, so she can't be pregnant."

I waited for her to cool down and said, "Okay, let's presume the ultrasound is wrong so let me examine her." This would give me an opportunity to question the girl and settle the matter temporarily.

As soon as the elder sister and her husband left the room, I asked the young girl if anyone had touched her. "No," she said.

"You have to tell me or I have to send you to a big hospital." I hated to scare her but that seemed the only way I could reach the truth.

"Bhaiya comes into my room to touch and cuddle me."

"Who is Bhaiya?" I asked very casually so as not to alarm her.

"That bhaiya," she said pointing towards the husband sitting outside.

"He told me not to tell didi as didi was pregnant," she continued in her childlike innocence. All this while the girl kept chewing the candy I had given her.

I called in the sister and her husband. Let me catch the bull by the horns, I thought. There was no other way and I was enraged. I looked at the sister and then at the husband and said, "It's him." He could not escape my direct gaze.

The sister could have slain me with her murderous gaze. The husband shifted uncomfortably in his chair. I could see beads of sweat forming on his forehead and he remained quiet.

"What a terrible doctor!" she snapped at me as she stomped out of the clinic. I never saw her again. I was amazed that she showed absolutely no sympathy for the little girl. Her reaction was to protect her husband. The sister could be sacrificed. Were we even human?

After all these years, I wonder what happened to that sweet little girl. Her body was too delicate and underdeveloped to withstand the abortion of a five-month baby. Moreover, it was illegal to terminate a five-month pregnancy. Maybe she bore it to full term, or perhaps she went to a quack and met her end there.

The young unmarried girls who entered my clinic with more than three months of pregnancy always faced the risk of losing their lives. Conducting abortions for over three months was illegal in India. Since the government had very strict rules for termination of pregnancy no qualified doctor would touch these girls; so they had no choice but to visit those dingy, dark clinics that had unscrupulous doctors or quacks who carried out even full-term abortions. No one knew how many of these girls died from these illegal abortions. The quacks were safe and smug in the knowledge that the parents would never utter a word about the shame of the daughter's pregnancy to anyone.

It was impossible to remain untouched and unmoved by these wretched incidents.

Girls as young as two years old were brought into my clinic with urine infections, sore and bruised private parts and unidentifiable cuts and bruises. I knew what had happened, but I was helpless and powerless. Talking to mothers and grandmothers about the abuse the young girls were experiencing within the home was futile. They would glare at me and accuse me of breaking up their family. Their harsh words of condemnation distressed me so much that I frequently suffered sleepless nights. Although it was the men who committed the crimes, it was the mothers and grandmothers who were responsible for this malaise in our society as they protected them in the name of family honour.

It was impossible for girls and women to report and prove that they had been abused as these acts occurred surreptitiously in the back seats of cabs, at workplaces, on buses, within marriage, outside of marriage, homes and every other place imaginable.

Let me just focus on the sexual abuse of young girls—it's a unique crime in many respects. According to an unofficial study, 67 percent of children in Delhi schools have admitted to being sexually abused at some point in their lives. Statistically, that means that two out of three children experience sexual abuse. Surprisingly, 40 percent of the victims are boys, so they need to be protected from sexual predators just as much as girls. The second unique point is that sexual abuse is the most hidden crime in the world as 90 percent of the victims do not report their experiences to anyone. I would go so far as to suggest that this statistic could be pushed to 99 percent with more studies and reports. Unfortunately, there is a code of secrecy and silence around sexual abuse, especially in children, for many reasons. Firstly, the child may not understand what has happened to him or her and, therefore, doesn't realise that it is wrong. Secondly, it's easy for a child to be coerced by the perpetrator to keep his or her mouth shut. Thirdly, sexual abuse is committed more often by the people the child loves, respects and looks up to rather than strangers. Consequently, the culprit is always sure that he will not be reported or caught. In fact, in India, the conviction rate is almost zero percent.

Lastly, it is unique because it is not a one-time act or a single incident. This abuse continues every single day for years and years until the poor child believes that it is a way of life. As a result, they are often left with no spirit to fight or resist, and they are scarred forever.

Most people believe that sexual abuse in children just happens to those who live in overcrowded slums, but that's not the case. After interacting with thousands of children, I discovered that sexual abuse happens across all socioeconomic strata of our society. We believe we have a good family structure in India, so why are there so many children who are sexually abused within the home? To help you understand the family dynamics, let me narrate a real case here.

A stately-looking old lady walked into the clinic one day with a three-year-old in tow.

"Please have a look at this girl, Doctor," she said.

"What happened?" I asked.

The elderly lady sighed, "She has trouble passing urine."

On examination, I noticed a bad case of infection.

"How did she get it?"

"When she was born," the lady replied, "the doctors did not clean her properly."

I prescribed a course of antibiotics and asked her to return in a month. I knew something was seriously wrong, but the clinic had been unusually busy that day and I thought I could do nothing about it anyway.

As she was leaving, the little girl looked back at me and the look in her eyes made me stop.

"Wait, can I please talk to her for a minute?"

"Why not?" said the grandmother with confidence.

I took the child back into the examination room and made her sit.

"Does someone touch you there?" I asked in a soft tone.

"No," the girl replied with haste.

Her response came a bit too quickly; I knew there was something amiss.

"You know, if you do not tell me, I will have to examine you with a needle," I said trying to put some fear into the child. I hated doing that but it was imperative. "That might be very painful," I added.

"You may even have to go to a hospital, so do not be scared of telling me. Let me see how brave you are." These fear tactics were the only way I could get the child to reveal the identity of the perpetrator.

Her eyes widened with fear, which made her mumble a name I recognised. "Gaurav bhaiya," she whispered so no one could hear. I knew that it was a deep secret she had been coerced to hide. "Gaurav bhaiya told me never to tell anyone or the police will take me."

"Why would the police take you?" I was taken aback at the ingenuity of the child abuser. This was a common trait amongst all of these depraved men. They transferred their own guilt onto the child leading her to believe that it was all her fault. In most of my counselling sessions, I came across even older girls of fifteen to seventeen years, who admitted to not telling their mothers about these hovering predators. "Why didn't you tell your mother if he was touching you?" I would ask. "She would never believe me," was one of the commonest reasons given.

"She would think that it was my fault," was another. It was terrible to know what little faith the parents and children had in each other.

Coming back to the little child who sat in front of me, I discovered that whenever her mother visited the neighbours or even went for a bath, he would quietly enter the room where she sat playing with her dolls and touch her. He had made her promise not to tell anyone about the little game they played and gave her a few sweets in return. The little girl started to believe that it was a little secret she shared with the adored Gaurav bhaiya. Her three-year-old brain told her that that's the way a family behaved.

When I came out of my room, I sent the child outside and approached her grandmother. "Who is Gaurav?"

"Oh, he is my grandson, her cousin. He is in college."

I informed her that he had been abusing the little girl. The grandmother was furious and her eyes shone with anger and agitation. She denied that anything of the sort could occur in her family.

"What are you saying, Doctor? We are not like this. Our family is very good, and Gaurav is a lovely young boy. He would never do such a thing. You do not know how respected we are, so please do not break up our family."

She called her granddaughter from the waiting room and started to yell at her. I could see the little child shrivel into herself as she wrapped her frock tightly around her legs.

"What did you tell the doctor? Who troubles you? Why are you lying? What did Gaurav do?" She badgered the girl mercilessly with her outburst.

I tried to calm down the old lady and said, "It is okay, do not be so agitated. It happens in lots of families. Just take care that it does not happen again. Please do not leave this little girl alone with him."

The woman strode out casting a furious look at me.

Two months later, she brought the girl again with the same urine and vaginal infection.

"Please write the same medicine as before; she became okay with it," said the grandmother in an uppity tone without meeting my eyes.

I wrote the prescription but could not stop myself from asking, "Did you take care of the problem?"

"Oh no, there is nothing like that, Doctor. She just made up the story because she was scared of you."

I have narrated this story because it is typical, and one can clearly see the family dynamics here. Numerous girls like the little girl have came to my clinic with similar stories—stories so similar that I could diagnose the problem as soon as they walked in either with their mothers or grandmothers. It was always the same righteous manner of the mother and the same subdued little girl. The world changed, the country changed, but this abuse remained the same. The perpetrator is always a trusted, well-liked and respected member of the family, but thanks to the mothers and grandmothers, he is certain that he will never get caught.

Hats off to the great Indian joint family! We are a patriarchal society, but every family has a Gaurav or a man in the household who can do nothing wrong. They all have an aura around them. How can a chit of a girl dare to spoil things?

To find out if children were suffering from abuse in affluent families as well, I visited a school in South Delhi.

"We have a good counsellor," the principal said to me upon my arrival. "Our children go to her, so they have no problems." She was a friend from school so I asked her if I could speak to them alone. From experience, I knew that in the presence of teachers the children would clam up and that would defeat the entire exercise. She allowed me to interact with the students as I wished, but added, "Our counsellor is good so I doubt that you will find anything worthwhile."

As the forty children huddled together on the first two benches, there was pin drop silence. I started by asking them two questions.

The first: "Statistics show that two out of three school children are sexually abused. Do you agree with me?"

One hand went up, then another, and then another. Soon 90 percent of the children in that classroom put their hands up.

The second question was: "Would you tell your parents or the school counsellor if you were abused?"

"Are you crazy?" one student said with amusement.

"No way," another replied.

"No way, Ma'am."

"What would you do instead?" I asked them.

"Phone a friend and manage it ourselves."

All the students in every class said the same thing.

"Why would you not go to the school counsellor?" I asked.

"The whole school gets to know even if you enter her room."

"Why not the parents?" I ventured.

One girl said, "I have an uncle who is in the army. He hugs all of us cousins and touches me in the wrong places."

"Have you told your mother about it?" I questioned.

"Yes, but when I told her she just said to move away after wishing him."

"Your mother did not say anything to him?"

"No, she said he would feel bad."

So, you see, we are sacrificing our girls to this big Indian family.

In comparison, Mumbai fared better due to the number of nuclear families and with more mothers who are working. Probably they are more aware of the problem. Girls are mainly abused by pizza delivery boys, liftmen, bus drivers and metro passengers, which does not make it any better, but at least they are safe in their family home.

Of course, the Principal was taken aback with my findings. She was thoughtful and quiet after hearing me.

I convinced her to install a locked letterbox in the lobby where any student could post any problem and ask for help. They could post anonymous messages and did not need to write their names, just use a password. I was happy to visit the school to help the students who dropped notes into the box. The system really worked. Almost every week, I received a call from the principal to come and meet the children who wished to speak with me and needed help. She allowed me to use a quiet room where students could come and talk to me in private. It was like Pandora's box that had been opened. Some admitted that older relatives had made sexual advances; some had faced harsh punishments by parents when they told them. Others had intrusive thoughts of suicides due to parental pressures, and some admitted to being gay. I helped many children just by lending an empathetic ear without being judgmental. I advised them and promised to follow up.

A few months later, I stopped getting calls from the Principal. When I called to ask what had been going on, the Principal told me that the parents felt uncomfortable about the whole letterbox thing and disallowed it.

I should have seen this coming as it is convenient to brush anything bad under the carpet. The malady is so silent and so insidious, that it does not disturb anything for anyone at all, then why create unnecessary hurdles? Denial is the keyword!